Hooves, muscles and sweat
The story of a pioneering Yorkshire equine physiotherapist

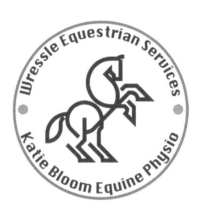

by

Katie Bloom

Foreword by Dr Jonathan F Pycock BVet Med DESM PhD MRCVS
President of The British Equine Veterinary Association 2017-18

Grosvenor House
Publishing Limited

This book is published by
Grosvenor House Publishing Ltd
Link House
140 The Broadway, Tolworth, Surrey, KT6 7HT.
www.grosvenorhousepublishing.co.uk

A CIP record for this book
is available from the British Library

ISBN 978-1-78623-516-9

Edited by Rupert Waddington (Executive Authors UK)

Front cover painting by the famous equestrian artist Daniel Crane.
It pictures from left to right the Blooms' three best horses
Ruby, Mr.Fielder and Mr. Cracker

CONTENTS

PREFACE..v
FOREWORD...vii
INTRODUCTION...ix

SECTION ONE - TWO LEGS..1
PART ONE – MADE IN YORKSHIRE..................................2
Chapter 1: Skylark – the Anglo-Polish Alliance 2
Chapter 2: All play and no work 10
Chapter 3: Rebel – with a cause..15
Chapter 4: Boys and biology 22
PART TWO – LEARNING THE ROPES (AND PULLEYS)....... 29
Chapter 5: Life beyond the Pennines 29
Chapter 6: This might hurt a little...34
PART THREE – DOCTORS, NURSES AND
SCRUM-HALVES 40
Chapter 7: The drive to freedom 40
Chapter 8: Carry on Physio - Episode 1
    (Hull Royal Infirmary) 45
Chapter 9: Carry on Physio – Episode 2
    (Goole Hospital) 50

SECTION TWO - FOUR LEGS.....................................57
PART FOUR – GOING IT ALONE 58
Chapter 10: Horse Wressling… 58
Chapter 11: "You're an equine what?"..................................66
Chapter 12: Working hard and loving it................................71
PART FIVE – EQUINE PHYSIOTHERAPY IN DETAIL 79
Introduction to Part Five...80
Chapter 13: The equine physiotherapy assessment 82
Chapter 14: The main problem areas 92
Chapter 15: Treatment and case studies 100

SECTION THREE – TWO LEGS *PLUS* FOUR LEGS............155
  Introduction to Section Three...............156
PART SIX: MORE FUN WITH HORSES 157
  Chapter 16: "Fools breed for wise men to buy" 157
  Chapter 17: Smoke and mirrors – buying and selling horses 165
  Chapter 18: Strutting the equine catwalk 170
  Chapter 19: The Sport of Kings (and some lesser sporting activities) 176
PART SEVEN – HEDGES, HOUNDS, HAUTE COUTURE AND HUSBANDS................181
  Chapter 20: Tally-ho! 181
  Chapter 21: In (and out of) the saddle................189
  Chapter 22: Glittering (sideways) from A to Z...............196
  Chapter 23: Posh frocks and politics – the Major and the Commander-in-Chief...............204

Editor's interview with the author 214
INFLUENCES and ACKNOWLEDGEMENTS 224

It is my contention that everyone has a tale to tell; every man or woman, regardless of profession or vocation. Moreover everyone with an interest in their friends, neighbours or community can learn much from the experience of others. Mrs. B leaves a small life window ajar for those who have an interest in horses, the horse world and the county of Yorkshire.

Take a peep through this window; it won't be time wasted.

Godfrey Bloom

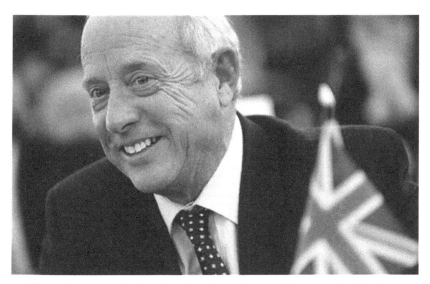

Godfrey Bloom, my husband, and without him pushing me, this book never would have been written.

FOREWORD

As an equine veterinary surgeon with a busy practice in North Yorkshire, I have known Katie for many years. For the most part we have had a good working relationship stemming from the mutual respect fellow professionals have for each other and their quality of work. Given the complexities of animal treatment, we've also had the occasional difference of opinion, but we have always respected each other's expertise and shared in common the best interests of the horse. And so it was with enormous pleasure when Katie asked me to write the foreword for her book as I was hoping it would provide me with some background and insight into one of the pioneering equine physiotherapists.

The book certainly does not disappoint. A neat blend of life story and the world of equine health in general, and of equine physiotherapy in particular, keeps the reader interested and stimulated. Of course the book is likely to appeal to those of us with an interest and passion concerning that most noble animal, the horse. The amount of detail is commendable and presented in such a way that it remains of interest to those with little working knowledge of equine veterinary medicine and physiotherapy.

Being involved in the world of equine politics, the relationship of veterinary surgeons and physiotherapists, along with other paraprofessionals such as equine dental technicians, occupies a considerable amount of time. By and large equine vets have a very good relationship with equine physiotherapists such as Katie. This is because they are professionals as we are. There is also a whole host of non-professional folks who believe they can assume a role in treating and caring for performance and lameness issues in horses. However, by working closely with the veterinary profession, it is the qualified equine physiotherapists such as Katie who ensure that the horse is the true beneficiary.

I congratulate Katie on managing what many of us aspire to, but never achieve, namely producing a book. Of course, this is only any use if there is an interesting and informative tale to tell. Katie certainly has such a tale, as you will find out by reading this well-crafted and fascinating autobiography of a true professional.

Jon Pycock MRCVS
2018 President BEVA

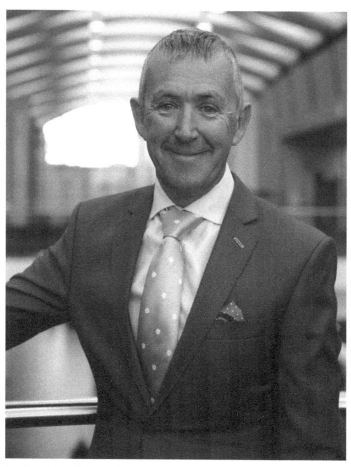

This is Dr. Jonathon F. Pycock B Vet Med PhD MRCVS President of BEVA 2017-2018 a friend and professional colleague who knows me well and has very kindly written the foreword.

INTRODUCTION

In one way or another I have dedicated my life to horses. And whilst that noble animal gives so many of us a shared interest, our understanding of the horse is far from a level playing field. In a way I have been lucky; physiotherapy by its nature requires an exploratory mind and keen observation. You never stop learning and your best teacher is often your patient. So I have had to question much that is otherwise taken for granted, and sometimes frankly wrong. I certainly don't have all the answers, but I do know that the horse world has still to appreciate the full potential of equine physiotherapy.

Now, when I first began to map out this book, I faced a problem. Godfrey, my husband, had generously suggested I write my life story; but I wanted to write a book about horses. And the more I thought about my experiences as an equine professional, the more there was that I wanted to say about my field of work and its relevance to horse owners, breeders, racers and so on. In the end I struck a compromise. I have written that autobiography, charting my journey from rebellious schoolgirl brought up in rural East Yorkshire to NHS physiotherapist and then equine specialist; but I have also slipped in extra chapters to share my passion for and experience of the colourful world of equine enthusiasts and professionals.

And on that note, you may be amongst the readers who spend as much of their time working with horses as I do and will already be very familiar with the equine explanations and descriptions. Please be patient with me! I hope there will still be something new for you, but my aim is also to reach those readers who may be less familiar with our world and yet will enjoy an appreciation of why you are so dedicated.

Before I begin my story, I want to make an appeal on behalf of the equine physiotherapy profession...

In all branches of modern medicine there is a trend towards relying more on technology to diagnose and treat. And today's veterinary care has some fantastic digital wizardry in its tool kit. But while this brings many miraculous advances in medicine, it also means that the proven benefits of traditional physiotherapy - working non-invasively with the body, prioritizing the animal's comfort, and even proactively involving the owner in the treatment as well as outcomes – can be overshadowed by the 'glamour' of modern techno-medicine.

Take a look at the definition of physiotherapy:

Physiotherapy: *The treatment of disease, injury, or deformity by physical methods such as massage, heat treatment, and exercise rather than by drugs or surgery.* (Oxford English Dictionary)

The key words here are *"by physical methods"*, treatment that begins with human examination and informed human instinct, two things that no digital or computerized machine can ever replace.

Vets today have to juggle different pressures – their own rising costs, owners who have 'googled' the topic and formed their own opinion, and even the ever-present threat of litigation if something goes wrong. But sometimes treating an animal needs to be a step-by-step process to allow different options to be explored. And in the case of, say, a lame horse, it makes so much sense for the first step to be physiotherapy for diagnosis and effective treatment. I have worked happily with many vets who confidently send me their referrals at the outset, knowing of course that if I find something serious or requiring veterinary examination the patient is referred back immediately. But sometimes there is a tendency to go straight into expensive, lengthy and ultimately unsuccessful treatment options before, finally, suggesting physiotherapy.

My NHS physiotherapy experience taught me the immense benefit of good interdisciplinary care models, with different professionals bringing their expertise to the table and collaborating to achieve a good outcome for the patient.

When both diagnosis and treatment are needed urgently, there is something wrong when we can't work together as a team and get it sorted out fast.

However, I'm not vet-bashing; I have immense respect for the profession, and I think in fact that we physios must ourselves take a little of the blame.

Despite unceasing efforts in the past several decades to educate the horse fraternity, we clearly haven't finished the job. There is still a lot of ignorance about the role of physiotherapy in understanding and treating equine problems. And even after we successfully achieved an amendment to the veterinary code that should have put animal physiotherapy in the mainstream of standard practice, far too many professionals still have little or no idea what we do – and what we can deliver; nor that it comes at a fraction of the financial cost and often the horse's welfare cost too.

To help address all of this, I decided to include in this book a sizeable chunk about the essential role of simple equine physio- therapy – soft-tissue manipulation and massage, and carefully designed exercise rehabilitation programmes. Ours is a profession that still needs all the help it can get to become better known and valued.

Animal care of any kind has moments of intense sadness but if you know where to look, it's packed with joy and laughter too.

And I would not trade a single day of my sometimes frustrating experiences as an equine physiotherapist if it meant losing just one of those joyful moments. I hope you enjoy sharing them with me in the pages that follow – and maybe gain a new appreciation of this valuable contribution to horse care in the 21st century.

CONTAINS:

Part One – Made in Yorkshire
(1961-80: ponies, cafés and schools)

Part Two – Learning the ropes (and pulleys)
(1980-83: college life and physiotherapy training)

Part Three – Doctors, nurses and scrum-halves
(1983-91: first physiotherapy jobs, Hull and Goole; exploring equine physiotherapy)

PART ONE – MADE IN YORKSHIRE

Chapter 1: Skylark – the Anglo-Polish Alliance

…Toby, the shetland pony that I used to cover in bandages…

…sipping cherry brandy when ill with chicken pox…

…the smell of old carrots boiling on the tack room stove…

…being bucked off a water-loving pony into ditches and puddles…

…ugly non-stretch jodphurs;

These are just a few of my most distant memories from my early years growing up in North Yorkshire. Memories? Some forty years later I'm still here, living in North Yorkshire, and still mucking around with horses! And that's not all that has remained unchanged.

Like many little girls who spent as much time as possible outdoors, I was a bit of a tom-boy. I dressed the part too, busying around our stables in drab workaday clothes that modern equestrian fashionistas would never dream of wearing. And today it's very much the same – I sometimes think I must keep our local charity shops going. But it's not laziness or a lack of appreciation for fashion – I do have a feminine side that just occasionally comes out on top. No, I think it is more a reflection of the solid, purposeful and common-sense upbringing that was my parents' greatest gift to me; an upbringing that taught me that life will knock you down, and you need to be ready to get right back up again. This gave me a determination and a sometimes foolish bravery that has stuck with me ever since, and that I like to think has helped me to lead such a rewarding career.

So, lets start with my parents.

My dad was an entrepreneur. From bookmaking to abattoirs, seaside cafes to riding schools, he seized whatever opportunities came his way to work hard, make a good living and enjoy life. He was also Polish – Richard Skowronek (meaning 'Skylark') – although because no one could pronounce his surname, it was his christian name he gave to some of his enterprises. I remember the bookies – Richard's of Howden - with the catchphrase, "Civility with Security"; only, thanks to his marked Polish accent, people learned this as "Servility with Security". Ironic, really, as servility was one thing my father never asked from anyone, and being a gambling business, security didn't really come into it either.

The catchphrase is important, though, as it reveals his sense of right and wrong. One day, for example, he was playing cards at the local hotel bar – he'd go down after work to let off some of the day's stress – and he found himself playing, and soundly beating, a miserable old Yorkshire farmer who drunkenly wagered his entire family farm on the game. Dad had been through a very tough war and knew what it meant to be skint; he wasn't about to see even this mean-spirited and much despised man in the gutter and duly let him off his wager.

"Chicken Richard" was his nickname in those early Yorkshire years but, as I'll explain, this had nothing to do with his war record. Like many members of the Polish army he began the war fighting on the side of Germany but ended it fighting with the allies against the Nazis. By the end of the war most of his family had been killed but his mother refused to leave Poland. My dad, however, was demobbed over here, in Bradford. And although he spoke very little English, his war experience left this young man of 22 feeling strongly patriotic towards Great Britain, and he decided to stay. He took board and lodging with a pair of spinster teachers, Bertha and Minnie Singles, in what was then a rather upmarket part of Bradford (Manningham Road, now sadly run-down and a bit seedy), and quickly found work at the town's abattoir. And the name "Chicken Richard" was simply an affectionate reference to his hard work in the immediate aftermath of the war at the abattoir and soon after running his own poultry and game business. Dad had in fact considered changing his surname to an English one, but my mother put her foot down; "You should be proud," she told him. And I think he was, both of his Polish heritage and of becoming a successfully-integrated member of England and, in particular, of Yorkshire.

So Dad was an industrious and a self-made man but with a strong sense of responsibility too. And I will never forget an example of this from the time I left school to study physiotherapy. I was eligible for a grant and so this was the first time Dad had not had to pay for my education. And I remember him saying: *"When you're qualified you're going to work for the NHS for many years to repay the good education you're being given for nothing!"* Not for him any free-loading!

I'm just as proud of my mother – and only too aware of how close I came to never being here! Mum nearly didn't make it to adulthood, suffering from tuberculosis as a child, the same illness that killed her two sisters. Her own father, my Grandad Long, had died while she was still a child. Having been a proud Royal Horse Artillery Sergeant who had fought in and survived World War One, he had gone on to work in the police and fire service. And it was in this civilian role that he was killed by smoke inhalation when rescuing some children from a fire. For this he was given a posthumous citation and the service helped to send my mother to school in Harrogate.

And digging out this photo of Grandad Long, I came across another one I must share with you – my Great-Grandmother (on my Mum's side) – Grandma Reilly. I never met her but I remember gazing in wonder at the picture of this formidable-looking woman in the Edwardian hat and listening to Mum's stories of being sent out to the shop to get her a fresh quart bottle of rum – one every day.

Following Grandad Long's death, Gran soon remarried to another policeman who we called Uncle Tom. We didn't like Uncle Tom, a judgement later shared by Mum when she discovered he used his fists to take out his ill temper on my Gran. Sadly I can't remember much about Gran except for one comforting image, a glimpse of her dozing by the fire in a rocking chair, with a pair of Jack Russells nestled fast asleep amongst her enormous boobs.

When my parents first met, Mum was working as a receptionist at the Station Hotel in Goole. They soon married, much to the general interest of the community – it was the 1950s and marrying foreigners was not something that happened every day. Dad was a catholic and when their first child, my brother Richard, came along their intention was for a catholic christening. However, having traipsed down to Howden RC Church to see the priest only to discover him blind drunk and incoherent, my parents decided that from then on the Skowroneks would become an Anglican family.

Soon after beginning work at the abattoir, Dad's entrepreneurial spirit kicked in and he set up his own business dealing in game and chickens; he'd slaughter and dress the meat and sell to restaurants and butcher's shops in the area. He loved this work, using his butchery skills first acquired in Poland before the war, being his own boss and developing a business reputation on his own patch. And by this time he'd moved out of the posh spinster home and was living independently in hotels, renting outbuildings for his business.

However, with a young bride and talk of children, he needed a family home, and so the family with the unpronounceable name moved to Howden, about 45 miles from Bradford. Dad had already acquired a workshop there, in Vicar Lane, followed now by a house in Knedlington Road and then a shop in Howden where he sold his own meats, sausages, cooked chicken and game. In almost no time at all, Dad had gone from abattoir worker to small empire builder.

Was my parent's marriage a happy one? I think so; they had the occasional row but don't all couples? The trigger was usually something about the business and although heated their tiffs were often comical as well. Dad's typical reaction was to take out his frustration safely on whatever lay near – I can still see him kicking over an enormous vat of dog food he was cooking, hot scraps and gravy flying all over the floor. One day Mum, driven to extremes, went as far as to throw a banana at him. I expect us kids just laughed. I do recall walking to a solicitor's office with her – but it was more of a gesture than of serious intent. So no, I think they were affectionate and they respected each other as equals. And that was a big part of Dad's attitude to life; even if you're the boss, you should treat everyone like family and ensure they're comfortable and content.

*

I came onto the scene in 1961, three years after my brother. And if not born actually in the saddle, I quickly made up for it and was caring for horses almost as soon as I could walk. Those early days also revealed evidence of the caring and nursing side that would eventually translate into my work as a physiotherapist.

Dad was a keen horseman; he'd talk about the old days back in Poland when horses were the main form of transport for many people, an everyday work horse during the week and then cleaned up for pulling the little family cart to church on Sundays. In the years ahead he was to embrace and share with me the English love of equine sport, especially hunting; but first we had to get some horses.

The house in Howden was semidetached but came with several acres of land behind it as well as some useful outbuildings, including a carriage shed with a granary on top and two stables. Dad quickly saw the potential, added a couple more stables, and soon I was having my very first encounters with horses right there outside the back door.

The first one I remember was Toby, a small brown and white skewbald Shetland pony. To be honest, being only three or four at the time I don't recall very much but I do know he had a placid nature that helped me to fall in love with horses. He would stand there happily without complaining while I systematically bandaged him from head to hoof like an Egyptian mummy – if only some of my human guinea pigs at physio college had been as patient! Bless him.

Soon after buying the house, Dad launched one of his ventures, this time a riding school. And of course, as soon as I was big enough I got to ride all of the horses – such a treat! I remember six of them, each with their own characteristics: Ruskin (a good horse), Gemini (a bucker – see below!), Molly and Pauline (both so lazy), Pedro (stubborn) and Rainbow Rocking Horse (a cheeky Apaloosa). It was another fantastic experience for a young child, to be able to learn first-hand that every horse is unique with its own personality and its own handling needs.

Gemini, an adorable little New Forest pony, had been my first 'real' pony when we still lived in Howden. However I'd had to share him with my brother Richard. And I wasn't very good at this. I remember a stand-off one day when I dug my heels in and refused to let Richard ride when he came home from school. My dad's solution was also a cunning way to teach me a lesson; he made me go out alone on Gemini and ride until sundown. Great, I thought! There was hardly any traffic in those days down the lanes, and so I happily hacked from home in Howden to meet up with Randolph Greensmith, my father's groom (the rendez-vous, his little apartment, was always known as 'Randy's Flats'). From there, with Randy accompanying on his pushbike, I rode on up the road towards Mr Faulkner's farm at North Howden. With lovely fields to ride in I was having the time of my life. But my God did I pay for it the next day, barely able to walk, much to my brother's amusement. Dad was no fool!

As a first riding pony I couldn't have wanted more from Gemini; he was a great teacher even if his methods were ungenerous and sometimes a little painful. You see, Gemini loved bucking. And because I was still small and relatively light, it was easy to be unseated. So, one moment we're trotting comfortably; the next, Gemini spots some tasty grass, bends his neck down to reach it – and if prompted to move on he would playfully buck and I'd go flying over his head. In the end we got him grass reins, designed to prevent the head going all the way down. But he was also a great one for refusing fences – another guaranteed way to hurl me off. The headaches and rattles in my skull that I used to suffer! But my dad always said; *"Don't tell your mother or she'll stop you riding. Just get back on and keep going."*

Little girls love messing around with horses, and once I outgrew my bandaging fetish I was able to explore the basics of proper horse care. I was always fiddling around with Gemini, learning about tack and bits, brushing down and so on. I think these early experiences can really help to seal a life-long love of horses; and I'm grateful to this day for having Gemini to teach me so young about the subtle dynamics in human-horse relationships.

*

Sadly but inevitably life wasn't just about ponies. There was also school which, until I was eleven, was the local junior in Howden. But I think they were happy days, apart from the shame of being chauffeured to school in Big Bertha, Dad's old Austin Comma van. I remember having some good chums to knock around with; and I used to get into a healthy amount of trouble and get my knuckles duly wrapped. There was one occasion when, thanks to the pre-Health and Safety playground era (no soft-surfaces beneath the equipment) I did both myself and my dignity some serious damage. I'd been swinging enthusiastically from the bars on the climbing frame, having a merry old time, when one of the boys called out: *"'Ey, I can see yer knickers!"* I instantly let go with both hands to pull down my skirt. Result – broken right elbow, broken left wrist, and two cut knees.

Although my life was mostly outdoors in the countryside or the yard, looking through some old photographs reminded me that as a pre-teen I wasn't entirely a tom-boy. Dad and I used to love sitting down together to watch 'Come Dancing' on the TV. I would pester him with comments and questions cunningly designed to elicit presents: *"Oh look at that dress, Daddy!" "Aw – I'd love to have a dress like that!"* I think he enjoyed seeing this more feminine side in his daughter – but it didn't manifest in a growing collection of gowns. For that I had to refine my technique further, many years later, and use it on a completely different target, my husband Godfrey.

But more about that later. For now, let's move on to a big learning curve I encountered at a tender age – the value of hard work…

"You lived in a shed? You were lucky! We had to put up with a cardboard box..." I wonder if you recognize those lines from the famous Monty Python TV comedy sketch, 'The Four Yorkshiremen"?

Well, it only came to my mind just now because I was about to compare the strenuous demands of my childhood with that of today's molly-coddled youngsters. But then I realized that I don't think any generation of children since last century have had it as tough as they do right now. How else do you explain the depression and general unfitness they seem to suffer? For me, growing up in the sixties and seventies, I had much better fortune – real, not comedic. And ironically some of that fortune came in the form of sheer hard work.

Yes, as the sketch says, life in the past was always simpler. But it was also a much safer and better place to learn as a child – so let's just go down memory lane to get some perspective. We had no social media, there were only three channels on the TV and no video recorders, schools were stricter, nothing opened on a Sunday... I could go on but the comparison is clear. So is the advantage that we had back then; we had to make our own entertainment or, as often in my case, it was found for us in the form of chores and jobs. And we didn't mind, not at all.

A busy and active child is usually a contented child. It's what nature intended, that children be continually learning from their experiences – and the easiest learning happens when they're not aware of it. A child needs opportunities but they can be really simple – a place to build a den, a tree to climb, a bird with a broken wing to nurse, a dog to walk. If it's fun or completely engaging, the child is happy. And if it reinforces learning – anything from simple numeracy to social interaction – so much the better.

And so it was for me and my brother – little wonder given my father's own tough experiences and his ceaseless entrepreneurial energy. He and my mum made sure we did not have time to be bored or inactive. As well as nurturing our own interests, we were expected to take an active role in family endeavours too. One I have particularly fond memories of is the café in Bridlington.

Not content with just running his poultry and game business and a small riding school, Dad decided it would be a great idea to add a small eatery to the business empire. And so he bought a seaside café that he ran during the holiday season, opening on Easter weekend and closing at the end of September. Mum was pregnant with me at the time and, as they were still living in Howden, there was now a 45-mile commute to fit into each day as well.

The Chicken Grill, as it was known, was a great success thanks to another of Dad's inspired decisions. He installed rotisserie ovens, a novelty back in the 60s, and the sight and aroma of plump chickens roasting throughout the day ensured a steady supply of salivating customers. But it was hard work too, so as soon as Richard and I were old enough, we were roped in to help during school holidays. Dad would drive us to Bridlington in his old Austin Princess, a huge whale of a car with a wallowing ride that always made me travel sick. Fortunately the café came with a small flat on the first floor and sometimes we'd stay overnight which added to the sense of adventure. But from seven in the morning I'd be helping out in the kitchens, and then from ten it was front of house duty. Hard work, but I was busy, I felt useful, I was getting really good at mental arithmetic and was generally very happy. I was even trusted with the job of staggering to the bank with each day's takings, large bags brimming with coins. I never grumbled because I never saw it as work, just something we all did together.

I continued to help at the café until I was sent off to school, as my brother had been a couple of years earlier. I don't know if anyone was hired to take over our duties, but I do recall that several years later Richard, now in his late teens, continued a somewhat on-off role in the business – and with all of father's enterprises. He hadn't been especially happy or successful at school, and Dad was a typical father with over-ambitious expectations. Theirs was a stormy relationship at that time, and my brother was forever being sacked and then reinstated – and then sacked again.

I should say a little more about my brother who I love dearly. As childhood siblings we had little to do with each other beyond the usual bickering. Richard was, however, excellent at seizing the upper hand when opportunity presented itself. I remember one Christmas day when, having fallen out with each other before lunch, he grassed me up to Mum and Dad after I gave him the V sign through a crack in the door. To this day we love repeating Mum's chastising phrase, "Not on Christmas of ALL days!"

It was his relationship with our father that I remember most, a difficult and sometimes stormy one as Richard approached adulthood. He had been a very keen sportsman at his school, Giggleswick, and not being especially academic he decided to follow through at college, taking meat industry and hygiene courses so that he could play a major role in the family business.

I expect any business that puts family members in close proximity every day can be inflammatory, and Richard seemed to annoy Dad quite easily. He had continued to play rugby after school, and had to take some time off work when he inured his ankle. Dad was very cross, I remember, and told him to give up rugby. Richard is a quiet person, not the type to pursue a fight unnecessarily, so he acquiesced and ploughed his spare energies into riding and hunting instead. But sadly even this had to give way eventually when the business pressures mounted.

Dad loved his son but I think could be almost cruel to him at times. I remember one incident a few days before Richard's wedding. Dad had been having one of his occasional bouts of childishness during which he generally fell out with everyone except me. I knew there was some kind of friction between them both and decided to go with Dad for a ride. I was married by this time and had more than enough confidence to stand up to Dad when required, but preferred to do it in the countryside on horseback if at all possible.

Eventually Dad turned to me and said: "You know, I don't think I'm going to go to Richard's wedding." So that was it; that was what had been brewing away and had matured into this ridiculous petty gesture, one he'd regret for the rest of his life. I remember leaning across from my saddle and grabbing him by the front of his shirt. "Don't you dare be so stupid and childish!" I yelled. "Of course you'll be there!" And I'm happy to say that he was, proudly watching Richard marry his bride, Jill Strangward, herself from an entrepreneurial family although this time in market gardening; and I swear that Dad's behaviour actually improved ever so slightly from that day on.

Back to the story, and to horses. When not preparing and serving chicken dishes, I was back at home where I took every opportunity to be working with the horses. My memory is of being an invaluable assistant to Dad's groom, Randolph ('Randy') Greensmith although I suspect the truth is that I spent most of my time with my own pony, Gemini. But I enjoyed Randy's company and must have absorbed a great many good techniques from watching him work, not least his dedication to the horses.

Randy was groom and gardener and general odd-job man. He was also a regular baby sitter so, one way or another, I spent a huge amount of time with him. He must have been in his late fifties and to me was huge, at least six feet tall, always standing very upright and projecting a handsomely large nose. A real traditional character and a good natural horseman, Randy's usual working wardrobe included voluminous woollen jodphurs, black hob-nail boots and woollen gaitors up to his knees, and always with shirt, waistcoat and tie, all topped off with a flat cap. For down-time on a Saturday night he'd announce to us that he was off to 'chapel'

- the local pub where he'd sink a few beers. But during the week he'd retreat, with me in tow, to the little tack room where we'd light the stove to keep warm and I'd be put in charge of carrot-boiling duty.

This routine of play and work all mixed up together would eventually mature into a work ethic that has really helped me through the years. As a dedicated student, then a junior hospital physiotherapist and finally as my own boss responsible for my business, I know just how useful it has been to find hard work both natural and rewarding. Of course there are days when I just want to be inside by the fire with the dogs or out fell-walking with Godfrey; and who knows, maybe I will be able to slow down the pace a little before too long. But I can't help thinking that it explains the malaise of today's youngsters who are not given similar opportunities – who are not pushed head-first into an exhausting but satisfying little tasks where they can grow in confidence and learn some useful life skills.

Of course, strip off the rosy-tinted specs and I have to admit that mine was not entirely a fairytale happy childhood – whose is? But a little hardship and discomfort can go a long way in building a strong backbone. And so I guess I should be grateful for the shock that was awaiting me when I outgrew junior school. But try telling that to my 11-year old self! I was about to be packed off to school – girl's boarding school – and I expect that by now you will realize this was not going to be an adjustment that I would find easy.

It's almost compulsory, isn't it, for a teenager to hit a rebellious phase? Well, I certainly struck my non-conformist high-point in my mid-teens, but for me it was in a positive way that has stayed with me ever since. And to this day, if I believe something I will say it openly; more to the point, if I believe that something's wrong or pointless I'll say so. If this pitches me against the popular flow then so be it. But I always have a reason for my belief – a 'cause' to underpin my minority viewpoint. I think the foundations for this can be found in these school years that oversaw a transformation from pre-teen tom-boy into serious young adult, and courtesy of two very different school experiences.

*

It was as a young girl out hunting that I'd first spotted them in the distance, a happy gaggle of neatly presented miniature ladies wearing red cloaks. I commented on how nice they looked and, somewhat rashly, how much I'd like to be one of them. My wish came all too true when, aged eleven, I left home to take up term-time dormitory digs at Queen Margaret's School for Girls, with my very own red cloak in my trunk.

QM's, as it's popularly called, is in Escrick, only a few miles from Wressle, but to me it was a world away from home. I need to say right now that today's QM is completely different to the one I got to know. In the past few decades all boarding schools seem to have undergone total transformation as they've strived to offer home-from-home comfort. But back in the nineteen-seventies, boarding school was anything but homely. In fact, to many of the old retainer teachers at that time the chief purpose of offering an education away from the home was to provide a character-building antidote to all that cossetting and comfort.

I should also say that whilst I may not have a great many happy memories of the red cloak days, I wouldn't go back and swap QM for somewhere else, no way. It's pretty clear to me that much of my determination and independence was molded during those five years from 1972 to 1977. And that independence kicked in the moment I was dropped off on my very first day.

Having unloaded my trunk from the car, Dad whisked Mum away so that I wouldn't see her crying. Public displays of affection were not normally a trait of our family, but this occasion would be too much for her. I wouldn't have cried anyway – being kicked, jostled and bucked by horses, and then being told not to blubber but just get on with it, had given me a determined stiff upper lip. In any case, there wasn't time to cry. As pairs of downcast parents drove away, we were bustled into small groups of eleven year olds, some sobbing, others like me looking around warily, and were then led off by senior girls to find our dormitories.

My dorm was in Queen Margaret's Lodge (now the Parsonage Hotel), an elegant but sprawling Edwardian lodge. The dorm was called Hyacinth, a small room with five hospital-style beds, each with horsehair mattresses. When I was researching this chapter I decided to take a little trip to the hotel to see if I could identify any former 'crime scenes' or recall the midnight feasts and other 'jolly japes' that we got up to. I found myself in the public bar and couldn't for a moment see anything familiar at all. Then it came it to me. This room had been called Delphinium in my day, a seven-bed dorm and just as cold and damp as Hyacinth had been. What I recognized was the large fireplace, now hosting a log-burning stove. Back then there had been a wooden cover over it; and I smiled, remembering how we used it to pull it across to hide some of our tuck box rations and tit-bits saved from school meals.

Each year we moved to a new dorm. One, Cornflower, sticks in my mind. With only four beds it was small but with just the right layout for some post-curfew fun. Once the lights went out at night, we'd dare each other to circumnavigate the entire room without touching the floorboards or carpet. We had to do this silently, and of course in complete darkness. Being quite sporty and competitive I was always up for this kind of thing; but on one occasion, having almost completed the circuit, I lost my balance and fell against a tall chest of drawers, sending it crashing onto the floor.

In came Matron; and out went Katie to spend an hour standing alone on the freezing cold landing. Not for the first time, nor the last.

The school classrooms were very traditional: wooden desks with tipping seats attached (and storage for all our books, as the teachers moved from room to room while we stayed put); ink wells in the desks (we all had to take turns as Ink Monitor – not even cartridge pens were allowed and certainly no biros); and all the desks were in neat rows and allocated carefully by the teachers to keep trouble makers far apart.

The classrooms usually had a raised plinth for the teachers' desk and chair so that they could tower over us menacingly. And behind was a rather fancy double sliding blackboard. Between lessons, if left unsupervised between the departing and arriving teachers, we'd sneak up and bang the blackboard rubber on the teacher's chair. Then, especially if the victim was our corpulent mathematics teacher Mrs Gerard, we'd try to suppress our giggles as she waddled off at the end of class with a fat, white bottom.

I remember one very grand classroom at the top of the front staircase; it was called the Glasshouse due to its stained glass windows and glazed walls. The pervading memory of the main building, however, is one many children from that era may share – the smell of cooking (boiling cabbage) mixed with wood polish, to this day a perfume laden with nostalgia.

My perception at the time was of school run by a coven of old 'Misses' who, I decided, clearly knew nothing about children. Instead of nurturing loyalty and affectionate respect, they seemed deliberately to promote a prisoner-of-war mentality in us. It's crazy if you think about it; why take dozens of hormone-riddled teenage girls and make their daily life an adversarial 'them versus us' challenge? Still, I'm sure some of my contemporaries have very happy memories and it certainly didn't do me any lasting harm. I did, however, hear from an old school chum who'd been back to a reunion event. There she'd run into a very old, frail lady on the front stairs who looked ashen and unwell. My friend asked if she was all right. *"Yes dear,"* came the shaky reply, *"I've just been putting a few ghosts to bed."* So maybe I wasn't alone in my perception.

A stark example of the lack of nurture was the occasion when, full of good intent, I put myself forward for the chapel choir. I'd had to climb up the steep steps to the organ loft in the chapel (itself pretty nerve-racking) to audition in front of the choirmaster. Now, I don't claim to be any good at singing; I expect my intonation lets me down (as it did each time I patiently tried - and failed - to tune my cello). But up in the loft I still gave a brave rendition of my prepared hymn, 'Dear Lord and Father of Mankind' - and was instantly and irritably dismissed. I didn't make the grade. However, not being in the choir did not mean you got out of singing altogether. Once a week all of us non-choir girls had to go to hymn practice in the chapel. Sopranos and altos were chosen according to physical size, not vocal range – so that made me an alto, no question! And one day I was standing there, giving it my best, when the choirmaster started wandering around and complaining that someone was singing out of key. Stopping in front of me he humiliated me before all the other girls by telling me to shut up. Needless to say I mimed from then onwards and to this day have no confidence in my singing, even in the shower.

In the early days I was an easy target for some light bullying. I was homesick and I'm sure it showed. But it was more my local accent that drew unwelcome attention. Try saying: "Can you pass the butter?" with Yorkshire vowels; it certainly amused two rather snooty older girls. Also I had a foreign name – and one that is

18

hard to pronounce – which is fatal when you're trying to blend inconspicuously into the background during lessons. And I was a large girl for my age, but that soon played to my strengths when I discovered a talent for lacrosse. Eventually I made Captain of our team, and fickle girls being as they are, this made me and my small group of friends the 'It Girls' everyone wanted to know.

From the first year at QM, I had my moments of being rebellious, but it wasn't just for the sake of it; as I've said it was pointless petty rules and disciplines that really got to me. And of course all schools, especially boarding schools for young ladies, rely on these to prevent anarchy. The teachers had a 'nip it in the bud' mentality, dishing out all kinds of ridiculously disproportionate punishments for the smallest of crimes. I recall wasting an entire afternoon outside the kitchens sitting with a bowl of grated cabbage salad and warmed stewed apple on my knee – Chef's Toe Nails we called this particular delicacy. I'd had a good go at it but just couldn't quite finish it; it was indescribably revolting, and as the hours rolled past became all but inedible. And even though I was missing lessons – no great hardship to me - I was still not allowed to move from the spot until it was gone.

Boarding schools have funny little routines that are either really irritating or become incredibly important landmarks in the slow passage of time before the next exeat or full holiday. Just a few come to mind now: Sunday evenings when the Head of House, Miss Hairs, would read novels to us while we sewed, knitted or made rugs; counting on fingers as we carefully made sure our pocket money books balanced (we were allowed five pounds a term to buy stamps, a few chocolates and pay for extra laundry); and Matron's ledger for ticking us off the bathing and hair-washing rota. One good thing about living in this kind of constrained environment is that you soon devise your own methods for avoiding detection when you fall foul of the rules. They should have called it 'initiative' and made it a formal part of the school curriculum.

Then I turned fifteen, and somehow it all changed. Did I become more of a rebel, or was I just growing bored of the same old routine?

It began with lacrosse; I began to get fed up with it and dropped out of the teams. I think I was also growing very body conscious; I was quite heavy set and I struggled to keep as fit as I'd been in the previous years. The lacrosse coach tried to motivate us but had rather cruel techniques; one tactic was to make us run a two-mile route in order to get our post. If you didn't finish it, no mail for you, and this was pre-mobile phone so letters were the only way to hear from back home.

This twisted carrot-and-stick strategy was exactly the kind of pointless nonsense (as it seemed to me) that I have always struggled to tolerate. I wasn't uncooperative just for the sake of it and I continued to work hard, but I also fought hard against cold spinster teachers and their silly edicts. And I fought hard on behalf of the weaker girls too; I've never been able to stand by and see someone bullied.

I did a few daft things – the ones everyone tries like smoking (for which I was gaited; and my parents were so cross that it calmed me down for a while). One fate I managed to avoid was suspension (or for some expulsion) for talking to the VBs – the local village boys – strictly forbidden but something that barely even occurred to me in any case. Eventually and inevitably, however, the young girl who'd been proud to wear the same red cloak as all the others was beginning to grow into a young woman who wanted to make her own mark. And so, like many girls in their mid-teens, I began experimenting with my appearance – with mixed outcomes.

First the ear piercing – I opted for the ice cube and cork method, and suffered the predictable septic consequences. Unfortunately they lingered long enough for my father to spot them on my next trip home – he was furious with me and chased me round and round the kitchen brandishing a metal bull ring. I swear he would have tried to insert it if he'd caught up with me. Then there was the startling red dye and perm. I can't remember what reaction this got, but perhaps my not remembering is because this time he decided to ignore it until it grew out – which it soon did.

What's really amusing is that for all his disapproval of my attempts at feminist emancipation, Dad was also up for conspiring in a few of our schoolgirl japes. In the fifth form we used to be allowed out for cycle rides. And one day I plotted with Dad to pick us up in the Land Rover just out of sight of the school gates and take us home for a slap-up lunch. To our shared pride school never found out. I'm glad however that he himself never found out about our post-O-level boozy midnight feasts around the school pool.

Was this 'rebel with a cause' in danger of becoming just a rebel for the sake of it? I don't think so. I was just doing the usual things that teens get up to it, testing the rules as I'd always done and searching for my own identity. But very soon I was to take drastic action to protect that newly emerging self. My next choices were going to be more about survival than appearances. The catalyst was that I was growing aware of how the school saw me and my future. And I didn't like it at all.

A handful of QM's cleverest girls from each year would be earmarked for Oxbridge entrance in the sixth form. But for the rest of us our destiny was not spires and quads; it was the Lucy Clayton Secretarial School or a cordon bleu cookery course.

I presented a problem. I was happy not to be eligible for the elite academic group, but I had earned a respectable eight O levels; and I was not an empty-headed fashionista ripe for marriage to an aspiring banker or a hereditary landowner. Nor did I have any interest whatsoever in cookery or becoming someone's P.A. My parents shared my concern about what I should do next, and fortunately my dilemma coincided with an emerging trend in private education – sending girls to boy's schools for their sixth form studies. And so I left Queen Margaret's and began a two-year stint as an honorary boy at Pocklington School, an old and respected former grammar in the Yorkshire Wolds.

Horses I understood, no problem; I'd almost been weaned in the saddle. And by now, girls as a species were no longer a mystery either. But boys? I still hadn't a clue about the opposite sex. My only real experience to date was of my brother, someone who taught me that boys existed to snitch on little girls and ride their sister's horses. However, in September 1977 this enormous gap in my human education was about to be filled as I joined fifteen other girls in a school of some 500 boys.

Why were schools doing this, introducing a tiny element of the opposite sex at just the age when both genders found each other particularly distracting? I don't really know, but it certainly provided a much-needed alternative choice for a great many girls in my situation. Having learned how to survive QM's I'd begun to tread water a little, lacking something to keep me sharp and motivated. It was easy to go home at weekends and school holidays and immerse myself in my ponies, in Dad's horse breeding and my great love, hunting. But if I was to complete the transformation into an independent adult with a good career I needed to be challenged once more. Pocklington was that challenge.

Beyond the Headmaster's house, a genteel ivy-covered Georgian building, most of the school was stark and barren and a far cry from QM's elegance. The main teaching block is a sixties building with huge and draughty iron-framed windows overlooking the windswept playing fields. Art and technology (and biology for some reason) were taught in chilly portakabins. And everywhere smelt of sweaty games kit and boiled cabbage.

To say that the school was not ready for girls would be an understatement. While the boys wore grey suits, white or blue shirts and black shoes, there was no uniform for us girls, just some rather vague and unhelpful fashion guidelines. And when the boys were enjoying a full range of sports twice a week, on Tuesdays and

Saturdays, there was nothing for us, no lacrosse or anything else – there simply weren't enough of us to make up a pair of competing teams. The one thing I was glad not to have shared with them was the corporal punishment; boys were still caned in those days.

We did at least have our own girls-only zone, essential for escaping the attentions of the bolder sixth-form boys and the doleful awkwardness of the younger ones. Our 'girls' common room' was in the Combined Cadet Force (CCF) hut, hidden away behind the main building. The girls' base had originally been in what became the Bursar's office, a small room in one corner of the main Assembly Hall. I expect someone in the staff room decided that this was too distracting to the nearby classrooms (and visiting would-be parents) and hence our relocation across the playing fields.

I began my Pocklington career as a day-girl, travelling a 34-mile round trip each day. But this wasted a lot valuable time and so we quickly changed this to a weekly-boarding arrangement with a lovely family, the Masons, whose son was also at the school. I liked them a lot and this solution made it easier for me to become immersed in school life but still go home on a Saturday to catch up with family and horses.

My first impressions were of just how clever the boys seemed to be. It was daunting after the lower academic bar I'd been set at QM's, but I soon got into the rhythm of the timetable and I put my head down and worked hard at my subjects – English, French, Biology and General Studies. The teachers made a huge difference too. Instead of the fussy and fusty 'Spinsters of Escrick' who prioritized ladylike conduct over exam results, I now had to answer to the scholastic demands of mostly male, often young and occasionally dynamic teachers. School life had suddenly become a whole lot more serious.

So I'd left the small and cosy world of Queen Margaret's as a belligerent naughty teenager, and suddenly found myself in a competitive and high-achieving environment. I knew I had no choice but to pull up my socks and prove the move had been the right one. And for my parents, having been told by QM's that for me A levels were pointless, I was determined to live up to the new expectations and do well.

We were a mixed bunch of girls. Some of course had one chief objective – romance. But I wasn't interested in getting a boyfriend. Once I got over the initial shock of all this testosterone and realized the boys were just people like me I made some good friends amongst them. Maybe it was the dormant tom-boy re-emerging in me? I don't know, but I was happy and really enjoying the different pace of life in a boy's school. I remember lunchtimes. At QM's it was all about good table manners and etiquette. At Pocklington it was all about getting the food down you as fast as you could as a swarm of locusts descended on grim tins of over-boiled potato.

One way or another I managed to stay out of trouble – almost. To celebrate completing our last A-level exam a group of us managed to sneak off to one of the small town's pubs, The Oddfellows Arms, and convince the landlord that we were of legal age. After too many pints of mild we then found a party to crash and the celebrations continued. All I remember after that was Mrs Mason hauling me home in the early hours. She was furious, understand-ably so being in loco parentis, and I wasn't proud. But I wouldn't have been me if I'd completed my Pocklington career without just one naughty gesture of independence to blot my otherwise accept-able record.

Then it was back home for a summer of horses and helping Dad – and waiting for the A-level results. And with them came a new problem.

*

During the sixth form – and one of the primary benefits of having upped sticks to Pocklington – we were encouraged to think ahead to our futures. To this day I'm not absolutely sure why, but I felt a pull towards some kind of physiological work; not necessarily physiotherapy but something that perhaps picked up where my earlier interest in bandaging dolls, Jack Russells and Shetland Ponies had left off. And so before sitting my A-level exams I had sent off my application to the University of Newcastle to read Physiology.

When the results letter came, I opened it. I'd failed Biology; so, no Newcastle degree for me.

Never one to let the grass grow, Dad immediately mapped out the next twelve months, what was now going to become my gap year: *"Don't think you're just going to spend the rest of your life here with the horses. You'll study and re-sit your Biology,"* I was told, *"and you can do some secretarial training, and work for me the rest of the time."* So that was that. And it was a good plan that kept me out of trouble but, of course, close to the horses I loved.

Studying for the biology resit meant two days a week at Hull Technical College. There I found myself being treated as an adult, and alongside other students who were also there voluntarily. After all those years at school it was refreshing to discover this new perspective – people who actually wanted to learn. For the shorthand and typing I gave up another two days each week, this time to a private school run by Dulcie Eggleston, a formidable teacher and lady. There was something timeless about the school, studying Pitman 2000 shorthand and typing to music to teach us rhythm and speed. It was great fun but I wasn't much good really; my heavy-handed pencil strokes were hard to decipher, and sometimes I began a typing exercise without checking my fingers were correctly aligned with the right keys, resulting in complete gibberish. But all in all this year of extra study helped to give me a sense of responsibility. I was growing up!

This year was also a time for some social growing up, if you can call it that. Pocklington had gone some way towards righting the imbalance in my worldliness after several years at a girl's boarding school, but it was the Young Farmers Club that gave me my first real taste of convivial socializing (and of serous boozing too).

Young Farmers clubs play many roles, one of which is to break down the isolation experienced by like-minded youngsters living in remote rural areas. So the social aspect was very important, and having joined my local club I seized the chance to become Social Secretary when the post became vacant. My duties included organizing a schedule of Wednesday evening events ('club nights') – anything and everything from farm walks, to visits to tractor sales rooms, factories, power stations and so on. And they always concluded with a visit to the local hostelry, then known as Sheila's Tavern (now the Barnes Wallis Inn). My brother was also in the Young Farmers, part of a group of extremely naughty boys, experts in all kinds of pranks and late-night mooning on the roadside!

Twice a year there were special Young Farmers events that brought different clubs together. One, the County Rally, was for all the Yorkshire clubs – and it certainly brought out the competitive streak in everyone. There were contests for all kinds of things - pork pie making, poultry trussing, trailer reversing, and even a fashion show. But once the prizes had been awarded the rivalry was soon forgotten in the drinking and dancing of the evening celebratory party.

Another event was the annual Young Farmers Conference. I only attended one, on the Isle of Man, but one was more than enough! I'm not sure that my liver has ever fully recovered from the volume of gin consumed in three days of parties and fun. And I can't actually remember much official business taking place; when not drinking we seemed to be forever engaged in water pistol fights. The shops in Douglas actually sold out of them, and rumour had it that one hotel was drenched on the upstairs floors, and mid-fight a vacuum cleaner found its way out of a bedroom window, assisted by a local and now rather well-known chartered surveyor... but I couldn't possibly comment!

I seemed to pack a lot of continued growing up into this gap year, but of course there was still the serious question to address: what was I going to do with the rest of my life? It was now urgently in need of an answer, and ideally one that made my biology retake a worthwhile investment.

At Pocklington I'd had the idea of a generalized physiology qualification that might possibly lead to something else, but now a lucky break led me in a more specific direction. Margaret Hunt, a friend of my mother, was a radiographer at the local cottage hospital in Goole, and very kindly pulled all kinds of strings to get me in on a day's work experience. I am eternally grateful to Margaret for this opportunity, something that in today's climate of litigation and health and safety would probably be much harder to organize. I enjoyed finding out what went on in a radiography department and it certainly ignited my curiosity about specific treatment modalities; but it also left me thinking that radiography wasn't quite what I wanted for myself. Once again Margaret led the way, suggesting a second day-trip, this time to the physiotherapy department.

Physiotherapy was run by a Mr Frank Oldridge who was blind but ably helped by Miss.Walduck, technically his receptionist but also very capable as a physio assistant (and as such a pioneer, as that post had not yet been invented). I was a little in awe of Frank and the way he moved effortlessly around his department; and I was bowled over to see them working with exercise therapy and electrical and manual treatments. By the end of the day I was hooked. Here was a career that combined my mummifying instincts with my wider interest in nurturing and healing, albeit up to that point only in animals. I felt certain that working with people would be just as satisfying. And so, at last, I had found my vocation.

However, it was still touch and go at this point. Despite Dad's efforts to keep me on task, I probably still managed to spend far too much time with the horses as, second time round, I barely improved my performance by only just scraping an E-grade pass in Biology. Fingers crossed it would be enough to unlock the door to my tertiary education. Applying to study physiotherapy meant applying to hospitals, but in the same way as the old university application system, with a short-list. On mine were Manchester, Sheffield and Cambridge and of these it was Manchester Royal Infirmary (MRI) that had offered me a place. However, their offer had been conditional on my getting at least a C-grade in my biology retake. But all was not lost. It seemed that the whole of the country was having difficulty that year in obtaining decent biology grades, and in this context my 'E' was judged adequate and I was accepted by MRI.

At last I was off on the big adventure of grown-up life away from home, and a chance to redeem my earlier academic record with the next few years of study and prove that I was up to the task I'd set for myself.

Devising safe routes from digs to college to avoid the Yorkshire Ripper; staying as far away as possible from the mass rioting in Moss Side; being squeezed into an unflattering leotard and expected to parade in front of my peers – these are just some of the challenges I faced during my three years in Manchester, 1980-83. I think the main test however, and the biggest success for me, was to consolidate the values and expectations I'd learned as a child with what the physiotherapy training now revealed about my strengths and weaknesses. And although I wouldn't realize it for a few years yet, this process was to help define my final destination, working with horses.

*

My god, I thought, it's Queen Margaret's and Pocklington all rolled into one! And certainly, if I'd chosen to go to the North of England's biggest city to enjoy student parties and freedom from rules and responsibility I would have been in for a shock. But fortunately (or was it naively) I hadn't left home with those ambitions. And when I saw how we were to live in the first year, I was glad of my QM's school experience.

First of all, our living arrangements: As a first-year student, I was billeted in a girl's hostel on Nelson Street. It was an intriguing location in many ways – opposite Number 62, the former home of Emily Pankhurst and the birthplace of the suffragette movement; conveniently situated next to the A&E department of the Manchester Royal Infirmary; and close by a huge car park where one of the Yorkshire Ripper's dead victims had been found. The hostel itself was a big detached Victorian house, with dormitories

29

and a communal kitchen. And, with iron beds, no cubicles to provide even the minimum of privacy, and a live-in 'Miss', our very own matron, it was just like being back in the school dorms.

One big relief for me, however, was the lack of petty rules (other than a strict ban on men). In fact, we were so busy, spending so little time there, that they just weren't necessary. Most of our meals were taken in the hospital canteen, so the hostel was simply where we slept and occasionally knocked together some food when there was space in the kitchen. We were treated as adults and were responsible for things like our laundry, although our student uniforms were strictly hospital property and never to be taken off site.

The work in that first year was intense and took no hostages; if you failed to make the grade you were out, no second chances. After a full day of classroom and laboratory work we had hours of homework to complete each evening. We were one very focused bunch of students, and compared to those on other courses at the Royal and at the university, we seemed to have no time at all for partying. Life in the five-bed dormitory in the hostel was very organized; two to three hours of silent evening study would be rewarded with a short spell of TV, and then bed. Weekends therefore became essential breaks from this intense routine. The other first-year students were mostly from Rochdale or Bolton, not far away, so it was easy for them to go home on a Friday. Not so easy for me, but by saving up every spare penny for my somewhat longer journey, I did the same, escaping on a Friday lunchtime to go back home, ride the horses and blow the city out of my lungs before coming back as late as I dared on Sunday evening.

Years two and three saw a big change when I decided to move out of the hostel and into rented digs with five other girls. We found a place, a typical Old Trafford Mancurian Victorian terraced house in Shrewsbury Street, Moss Side. However we must have been lucky in choosing our street, as all the only impact of the infamous riots was that we were unable to get to college for a day.

I'll always remember my move to Shrewsbury Street. At last we were fully-accredited independent grown-ups! And that meant supplying all kinds of things yourself, including a bed. My father had a big butcher's van, a Ford Transit, and one Sunday, with the entire family on board, we set off for Manchester. As we reached the city our route took us on a mini tour of some of Manchester's multi-cultural parts including the Indian area of Rusholme and the African area of Old Trafford and Mosside. This made quite an impression on my father who knew nothing of the city and, on their return journey, apparently kept shaking his head and asking: "Where have we left our Katie?"

As things turned out, brothers, fathers and boyfriends all warmed to our house as it virtually overlooked the Old Trafford cricket ground. But for us ourselves it meant freedom and the welcome absence of a Matriarchal authority figure breathing down our necks. In truth we were still far too busy to live it up much and enjoy the hedonistic student life. And of course money was as short as ever. Buses were a luxury so instead we would cycle or walk the four miles from Moss Side to an 8 a.m. start at college. And I remember how we used to dress in several layers of clothing of an evening so we didn't have to feed the gas meter. But we enjoyed the house, especially being able to share meals together and sit and talk about the course. And just occasionally we managed to treat ourselves to an evening out. I have fond memories of one of our group, Sue Leigh, with her Princess Diana hairdo and her skilled put-downs for over-attentive young men, who introduced this inexperienced Yorkshire lass to the nightclub scene.

I continued to go home to Wressle at weekends – thank goodness for student railcards! In the winter I'd hunt but at any time of year there was plenty to get stuck into – bathing horses, cleaning tack, even cooking the Sunday lunch. I'd also meet up with friends and go to Young Farmer's parties, and I even managed to find time for one or two fleeting romances. But every weekend ended the same way, the late Sunday afternoon trip back to the coalface.

Our studies in the second and third year of training was much more hands-on, typically a morning spent in college and then the afternoon on the wards or on placement at special units. And this is where I began to realize that there are two distinct styles of medical care – the care to minimize discomfort, and the care to treat and cure problems. As a physiotherapist your work easily covers both areas, but as I was to discover my vocation lay more in the latter, facing problems and resolving them, not just easing suffering or providing succor. I'm sure this goes back to childhood and especially to my dad's pragmatic take on life. The challenge and satisfaction of a diagnose-treat-cure process is irresistible, even when the final outcome is a compromise rather than a complete cure. I definitely need to see my patients up and about again, able to do much of what they could before. And of course, as time would tell, it's the same with the horses I treat.

What I knew deep down, however, is that even the most clean-cut and cure-focused treatment still requires a large dose of the same compassion that is essential for the more maintenance and palliative types of care. And in the horse world, where beasts have just a tiny fraction of the value that we humans enjoy, I think this has really helped me to persevere with a damaged or unhappy horse when the owner might just as easily have washed their hands of it. But I still need to believe that improvement is definitely possible; I still need to be working towards something tangible and better, however small.

It was an interesting time to be training in physiotherapy. The practice was still largely a prescriptive rather than diagnostic intervention; physios were told what the problem was and were then required to dish out the appropriate treatment. And of course, while working in clinical settings as a student, we had to follow the rules to the letter - I was to see a very different side to the profession once I began working as a qualified therapist in Hull. But this rigid training structure worked well. And it also gave me a chance to learn about the professional relationships that keep hospitals going and, we hope, help deliver the best care, something that would come back to me when I began working with vets.

Before sharing some of our student experimentations with treatments I just want to end this chapter by reflecting a little more on the evolution of the physiotherapy profession.

I left Manchester in no doubt that I'd had a very good and thorough training; there was no question about that. And it was delivered with the kind of robust thoroughness that has informed my work ever since – we had to learn everything about a condition, from signs and symptoms to the full range of possible treatments (drug, operative, etc). But being a prescriptive intervention, one of those treatment options, we were not actually expected to apply all of that knowledge; our role was just to pick up where the diagnostician left off. Yet even so a physio's work was still a bit hit and miss. Some techniques were novel or evolving and we were always looking for new ways to use what we knew and the tools that we had. You really had to apply your imagination and think outside the box sometimes. And of course this put me in good stead when I began working in equine physiotherapy, a new specialism that had barely left the starting gate.

So, I have always placed huge value on medical intuition and the opportunity to develop this in my training. And whilst today's students and qualified physiotherapists may have a much more comprehensive tool kit of remedies for specific conditions, I wonder if they get as much chance as we did to hone their intuitive skills? And with modern Health and Safety restrictions and the ever-present threat of malpractice litigation, are they able to use it even if they have acquired it?

It's a fascinating problem – just how do you rehearse an invasive and potentially painful medical intervention? At what point do you have to put away the books and start doing it for real, replacing theory with practice? And who will be your guinea pigs? Well, for better or for worse we did it this way.

Our college day was split in two, the mornings in class-based theory and the afternoons in the real world, watching and learning. In some ways, the toughest was the classroom learning – over one thousand pages of Gray's Anatomy to digest so that you knew every muscle insertion, attachment, action and nerve supply – and then the same for all the joints too. Alongside this we had to learn and understand all the different massage techniques, exercise therapies, electrical therapies and Proprioceptive Neuromuscular Facilitation (PNF), the latter invented by our then principal, Miss Pat Waddington).

However, the best way to understand anatomy is through hands-on learning. And we took two contrasting routes to achieve this. One was via the anatomy practical for which, modeling leotards, we would take turns playing the patient. And the merriment this caused proved an important tonic after the other practical learning route. You see, to understand how the body fits together, the ultimate route is by taking it all apart. So, alongside the statutory human skeleton (keen students bought their own and in those days they were real deal, not plastic imitations), we got our hands dirty examining human corpses donated to the dissection labs of the medical school on Oxford Road.

I can still recall the overbearing smell of formaldehyde and the cadavres in the inelegant stages of being dismantled. So yes, it was pretty gruesome, but it was also essential if we were to heal rather than maim our patients; and I suppose this experience is why some medical professionals become blasé about the body and can forget to sugar the pill when talking to terrified patients. For me, however, the lasting impact of dissecting deceased people has been to respect the ephemeral nature of life.

Our placements, on the other hand, were our opportunity to gain familiarity with different clinical settings and to begin applying some of what we'd learned, albeit under very careful supervision. But an additional and extremely valuable goal was to see how other medical professionals worked – including notoriously tough figures like Ward Sisters.

I remember one placement with a fellow student on a male neurological ward. The Sister was fairly typical in her dislike of physiotherapists, and with some justification. She would see them swan in to her domain and take over. Then, having usually had to cause discomfort or pain when administering their treatment, they could just swan out again leaving the nurses with the task of trying to soothe the disgruntled patients. So, faced with two students who were simply there to learn about the ward and its specialty, this Sister decided to inflict a baptism of fire. She set us the task of sorting out a new arrival, a filthy and fragrant tramp who, having suffered a stroke, had been found collapsed on a rubbish dump.

We put on our bravest faces but were both incredibly nervous as we went through the admission process and then began to clean up the poor old chap. Sister however looked on with a wry smile; remember, neither of us had ever bathed and shaved anyone, let alone someone in this condition. And she knew it. He was conscious and able to help us a little, and must have been exhausted himself by the time we'd finished. But we did it and we'd passed Sister's test; and she never hassled us again for the remainder of our two-week placement. In fact, as the days passed a caring and compassionate woman could be glimpsed behind all that fierce efficiency, something that made a huge impression on me and taught me to appreciate other professionals, however they may initially present themselves.

To learn about specific physio treatments we often had to use each other as guinea pigs. It's easy to laugh at it now but we could easily have done each other real harm. I wonder if today's Health and Safety police would allow this kind of thing to carry on at all? One that gave us great fun was Faradic Treatment, a rather primitive method for applying electrical current in order to get muscles to contract. There are much better forms of electrical stimulation nowadays, although I think they carried on teaching the old method until about ten years ago – it's curious how training sometimes seems to lag behind practice.

The faradic process was simple; for example, you might have a footbath with two metal strips in the water and attached at the other end to the faradic machine – switch it on and the result should be stimulated muscles and twitching feet. But the 'fun' came with its application for Bell's Palsy (facial paralysis). You'd position one electrode close to the facial nerve and use the other to stimulate specific parts of the face. And my goodness that could hurt! But you could get an easy laugh by making the student guinea pig's eyebrows go up and down involuntarily or their nostrils twitch.

Another one we tried on each other was shortwave diathermy[1], a heat-based muscle relaxing process. Under the guise of trying it out for learning purposes we would use it, with good intentions, on students who'd had painful or heavy periods – not something I would advocate nowadays!

That was in the mornings. Our afternoons, out on two-week placements, were more closely supervised. All of the treatments had one thing in common, to try to keep the body working as well as possible. And while many people think this means joints and muscles, they may be surprised by how we can also help with tissue damage too. I remember doing my stint in geriatric care at

---

[1] Diathermy that delivers local heat to various tissues via shortwave frequency electromagnetic waves.

Barnes Hospital on the outskirts of the city. There we had elderly patients who were mostly immobile, some with different degrees of dementia, and much of our work was treating the terrible pressure sores that would develop on their heels and bottoms. At that time there was little expertise in preventing these kinds of injuries and the sores really were horrific – you could easily get your fingers right in.

The physiotherapist we were observing worked really hard to heal these sores with a machine that used steam, ultraviolet, laser and sometimes ultrasound. I remember we used to feel pretty sick after using it! But you could really see the difference; where there had been black, smelly wound now it would be lovely and pink and healthy. And the physio would then pack the wound with gauze covered in cod liver oil honey or yoghurt.

Talking of 'that time', the typical 1980s hospital still looked a little like the film set for Carry on Matron – old-fashioned metal-framed beds, sheets, blankets and counterpanes (with meticulous 'hospital corners'), and very strict visiting rules. The rules for us were strict too – no sitting on patients' beds, absolutely no attendance during ward rounds (a good indication of where we fitted into the food chain - extraordinary to think that students were forbidden this rich learning opportunity), and all plants and flowers had to be removed and taken to the sluice overnight. Sisters ruled with a rod of iron, but they also ran extremely efficient and clean wards.

One placement I really didn't enjoy was in the hydrotherapy unit, a treatment loved by the patients but not by us. The therapy is simple and effective, a pool of warm water to help the patient relax and, with a little support from us and the water's buoyancy, the effect of zero gravity to take the weight off joints and muscle while we worked on the problem areas. But in those days the pools were pretty grim, especially if you had to spend half a day standing in the chlorine-rich water. We would work in swimming costumes, but these would rot very quickly in the chemical mix, giving you a good idea of how unpleasant it was. I think today's hydro pools are probably much better (a rare win for Health and Safety).

Finally, there was one placement, a school for children with severe disabilities, that really challenged me but in a good way. It was on the Cheshire border and I had to cycle to the station, take the train and then cycle to the school. We had actually finished our final exams but placements continued - and this one taught me a lot about myself.

The children had a range of chronic problems such as cerebral palsy. Some poor souls were so locked up by their disability that they were all but catatonic, and our main focus was to maintain as much physical mobility as we could.

I was particularly anxious of this type of work and environment; I found the children's predicaments very emotional and hard to accept. And as this work was more to do with preventing further physical deterioration rather than delivering a tangible improvement, it didn't resonate well with my primary interests as a physiotherapist. However, my supervisor was very canny and saw through all of this immediately. She knew that I needed to experience the environment and particularly to understand what motivated those who did work with the children, day in and day out, and with incredible dedication.

A lot of mums were regularly involved in the school, and watching them at work it was clear that they themselves were experts in their children's physical therapy, learning by assisting the school's excellent specialist physio. And of course, as they lived with this every day, very little shocked or traumatised them. A child might suddenly suffer an epileptic shock at any moment, but everyone would smoothly and quietly switch into response mode. This taught me two very important lessons – 1) when you know what to expect and exactly what to do, nothing need become a crisis; and 2) while the physio can diagnose the problem and decide on the treatment, you often also need the parents (or, in equine work, the owners of the horses) to be suitably equipped or trained to follow through.

These lessons have served me very well ever since, and are something I hope I have passed on in turn to my yard and physio teams.

*

It was now August 1983, and I had just passed my final exams. I was a newly qualified physiotherapist, and what a journey it had been. I felt immensely proud but also nervous as I applied for my very first physio job. I needn't have worried. It soon became clear that almost everything to date had prepared me well for what lay ahead. The real test would be finding the confidence and gumption to pull it all together...

We'll leave some of the more extraordinary treatment stories for the next two chapters – and with them a reflection on medical life before Health and Safety went into overdrive. First I'd like just to paint the scene – an NHS hospital in the 1980s, some of the influential people I worked with, and the extra-curricular activities I enjoyed (and no, they're not what you think).

I worked in the NHS for a total of eight years between 1983 and 1991, and could sum up that experience as a kaleidoscopic mix of hapless victims (the patients), inspirational colleagues (the gold dust of the NHS) and tyrannical bosses (the ones struggling to make ends meet). But one way or another they all helped to turn this nervous newly-qualified phsyio into a confident and innovative problem solver. So I thank them all.

*

Hull Royal Infirmary was some 30 miles from home, along pretty treacherous roads in winter; so first things first, I needed a car. As a basic grade physio, my starting salary only just broke the £5000 barrier. But I was a very lucky girl; Dad decided to celebrate my first job by buying me my own set of wheels, a Mini Metro 1100, dirt-brown in colour, registration A446 NKH, and with beige velour upholstery. I loved it and life was good! I loved the car; I loved the speed (getting up to the magic ton on a trip to the Lakes); I loved being able to whizz straight into the free staff car park; and I loved getting home by six in time to see to the horses. Of course I wasn't completely independent, still living at home and subsidized by my parents with free board and lodgings. But I'd made a start.

The hospital is in Anlaby Road, close to where Hull City Football Club used to be and not far from the Hull Rugby League Club. The main hospital building, at the end of The Boulevard, is an enormous broad 1970s block, some sixteen floors high. And my first memory of the job was attending the compulsory fire lecture. We were made to sit and watch a pretty gruesome contemporary video of a burning building in Sao Paulo, with people jumping out of high-rise windows. Well chosen! It made sure we paid attention and never forgot the basic fire precautions. In fact in the summer particularly you'd always glance up at the windows nervously as they were kept wide open, the south-facing building sweltering without the benefit of air-conditioning. It wasn't a great environment for people who were feeling ill.

As a Basic Grade (today they would be offended by this term, preferring to be known as Juniors) my quality of life was heavily influenced by my immediate bosses. We began by working on a three-monthly rotation scheme so that we got the broadest possible experience. And the first of these placements had me working mornings in the Outpatient Physio Department, and afternoons in the gym assisting with neuro/medical and surgical patients. This put me directly under three influential people and gave me a great opportunity to learn; while we were expected just to get on with the job, we were also encouraged to ask questions when we needed to. However, that wasn't always easy.

The senior physiotherapist in Outpatients was a woman called Alex Fuller. An experienced physio, she commanded tremendous respect from us, but she was not very approachable, quite frightening in fact. Alex was tough and rarely showed any outward emotion about the work or the patients; she was also economical on empathy towards new members of the team. If you did manage to find the courage to ask a question you were likely to get a reply laced with sarcasm. But I think in fact that she knew exactly what she was doing. Nowadays I meet up with Alex from time to time (we get on very well) and was recently recalling these days with her. I suggested that maybe she was sometimes a bit too tough; her blunt Yorkshire reply: "Well, you can't have it all handed to you on a plate; I wanted you to think and use your brain, to make you learn."

She's right of course, and she made us all work very hard for her. She makes even more sense when seen as the 'bad cop' half of the teaching team. The 'good cop' role was played by Geoff Plummer, a splendidly tall man who ran the gym-based physio, and his colleague Dr Gosnold who ran the A&E operation. Geoff was only a few years older than me but a tremendous motivator. He became a good friend too, and was a welcome guest at our thirtieth wedding anniversary. In their spare time, these two characters also worked for Hull Kingston Rovers. And, with all those fit rugger players to work on, I wasn't going to miss out when offered the chance to assist. So during some lunch breaks or after work I'd join them at the ground up the road. My total heartthrob at the club was George Fairburn, but it was another player, Phil Lowe, who I came across many years later. He had taken a pub close to where we live, and from across the bar he regaled us with memories of what a really hard taskmaster I'd been – hard to believe given what a tall, strong and intimidating figure he had been and still was.

I must have enjoyed this sporting sideline as I decided to offer physiotherapy help to another club. It was the team my brother played for and one that took me back to an earlier time, Pocklington Rugby Union Football Club. But what a contrast with HKR. There was no physio tradition at Pocklington and therefore no expectations of me, so I suggested that I could start by assessing their pre-training warm-ups. Warm-ups? They consisted of little more than the players extending their legs as they climbed from their cars still munching on their sandwiches, just one minute before training began. My attempts to demonstrate some stretching techniques were met with guffaws and ribald comments. And after just an hour of training everything ceased and they headed for the nearest bar for a liquid 'warm-down'.

However, they say that everything comes to those who wait, and sure enough I had my opportunity to shine – well, almost. I had accompanied the team (as official bag lady) to a match against Hull Ionians. There was a particularly nasty collision on the pitch and at last my moment had arrived. I ran proudly onto the turf clutching my equipment bag and an ice bucket – to much laughter around the stadium. Behind me I was leaving a Hansel and Gretel trail of unwinding rolls of bandage. I'd forgotten to fasten the bag.

Things didn't really improve and, a little discouraged, I left the club after two years. I think that things have changed since then – perhaps they were the last of the hard brigade! Today there is much greater professionalism, and they enjoy all the benefits of a permanent affiliated physiotherapist. I guess that in every new situation someone has to play guinea pig and put their dignity on the line. If that was me, I'd like to think that my antics and missionary work played just a small part in helping change hearts and minds.

Now, I really want to push on and talk physiotherapy, but there are just a couple of amusing memories of hospital life to share first.

There was some excellent team spirit – I think there has to be in these kinds of jobs; you know the saying; "you have to laugh or you cry". So, if you were ever down in the dumps there was always sanctuary to be found somewhere – like the staff coffee room for example on the second floor, although as it doubled as the smoking room (can you imagine that today?) you were advised to take some oxygen with you. The alternative, if you could wait it out until the end of the week, was the gang's Friday lunchtime visit to the pub, returning to their patients with beer on their breath…

Talking of smoke and breath - I'll always remember one character, Old Dot at the hydro pool. Dot was an auxiliary nurse and positively ancient. She dressed in a grey uniform that perfectly offset her scarlet red lipstick, and she chain-smoked. Her room was dense with lingering smoke and the acrid stench of fag ends;

and her breath... well, there was no escape for the patients as she helped them in and out of their pool clothing. But they forgave her because she was a real sweetie too, rather like Julie Walters' character in the TV show, Dinner Ladies.

And finally, there was one lovely tradition that brought everyone together whenever a member of the medical staff was leaving their post. Doctors, physios, nurses – they all received the same send-off, an embarrassing tour of the hospital strapped into a wheelchair, half-naked and bandaged to the hilt - and ending up at the hydropool for the ceremonial dunking.

Perhaps the funniest moments, however, were the unexpected ones when treating patients...

Nowadays, if you're referred to outpatient physiotherapy by your GP, you can expect thorough examination and then a going-home gift - some paper with instructions for some exercises, printed out from the NHS website. And no doubt this ticks lots of boxes and keeps the bean-counting managers happy. But in the 1980s we didn't have the advantage/disadvantage of the internet, and this affected not just the patients but the physios too; when confronted with an unusual problem we had no instant global resource to consult. So, as has marked my own practice to this day, we often relied on a huge dose of initiative. We also had more primitive equipment to work with. And this, together with much less of today's cloying safety culture, meant that sometimes things did not go quite as planned...

*

We were administering a routine treatment, shortwave diathermy, to an old man, but with a machine that should now be in a museum. The contraption used rubber pads inside double layers of felt with holes in it, all wrapped up in a kind of pillowcase, with an electric lead coming out of it. The idea was to apply warming shortwaves using two pads through the problematic joint or the back or neck, from front to back.

The physio in charge had applied the pads and left the elderly gentleman lying on the bed, drawing the curtain around him for privacy. After a few minutes I peered around the curtain to check he was comfortable – and saw smoke gently billowing from behind his head. As was all too easy to do, the pads had been incorrectly set up, reducing the crucial insulation between equipment and patient. Thank goodness we'd got one part of the job right, removing his hearing aid before we started to prevent the shortwave machine doing crazy things with it! There were no actual flames, so I quickly unplugged everything and wafted away the smell of burning rubber. Fortunately for us Alex Fuller wasn't around that day, and the patient was completely unaware of the problem; and, with no smoke alarms back then, the rest of the hospital was undisturbed too.

Afternoons were hard work, with patients suffering from strokes, head injuries or recovering from brain surgery. I remember a very sad case, a young farmer, a typical East Yorkshire type. He had suffered a left-sided stroke and, being very tall and lean and with his left side paralysed he had real difficulty retaining his own balance when sitting. His damaged brain gave him a misleading sense of where his body was in relation to the chair and so he overcompensated.

He was called Len, and he had a wry sense of humour. Coming from my own country background we soon hit it off well, which is always a bonus when you start manhandling your patients. I would first sit Len in front of the mirror and then gently push him this way and that so that he could relate his sense of his movement to what he actually saw it. *"Are you as rough with your horses as you are with me?"* he would ask me, grinning.

My own technique was still a touch embryonic and although I took great care I obviously didn't always support him properly – sometimes Len would keel over like a slow-motion felled tree and tumble onto the floor. With no feeling in his left side and laxity in the shoulder joint he could easily have dislocated it with the fall, poor man. He did make a reasonable recovery in the end, learning to walk again, but his arm movement was always going to be limited.

Gym work was always fun, especially as I got to work with the inspirational Geoff Plummer. In the mornings we'd deal with different categories of injury – early knee injuries, medium and late, foot injuries, backs, shoulders and so on. Geoff always made sure there was plenty of good hearted banter going on – team spirit to help patients through what could often be painful. In gym work you need your patients to do their bit, and as a physio you're always looking for new ways to motivate them. I remember one 'blonde' moment I'm not proud of. I was trying to get a group of men to do pull-ups against the wall bars – completely overlooking the problem posed by their male anatomy getting bruised and bashed by the bars.

Not all treatment was so physical, however. We also helped patients with soft tissue injuries such as bad cases of the skin condition, psoriasis. Back then these poor wretches would be hospitalized so that they could be wrapped in loads and loads of bandages, changed daily, and be bathed in horrible coal tar mixtures. Our input was to use ultra-violet light as part of their topical treatment. Now, these were big machines, nothing like today's neat sun beds, and they could burn you in seconds. So we had to begin with a small test to check the patient's response – a bit like fabric treatments today: *"test on an inconspicuous area before applying fully."* Our test involved a small piece of lint with three tiny holes in it that had to be held a small distance from the skin and the machine turned on for five seconds, ten seconds and so on until we reached danger point.

The machine was terribly inaccurate, so our judgement was crucial. And anyone in the vicinity had to wear protective goggles. Despite this we weren't really aware of the danger from UV light and, if we were about to go on holiday, would sneak in for a little self-application to get some extra skin tone.

Intensive care was the one department that did not bring any humour to the work. Here we were treating unconscious patients, with head injuries or coma, for example. And it's really important in this situation to keep the person's joints and limbs moving to maintain the circulation. Nowadays there are all kinds of clever devices like ripple mattresses, but before that it was down to hands-on interventions. Other physio roles included keeping the chest clear for patients on ventilators. You might also be called in to help when an unconscious patient's brain activity suddenly creates an area of spasticity in a limb that needed stretching out.

I found intensive care, and especially the neo-natal work, very tough going. It was partly the absence of repartee you enjoy with the awake patient, and partly the strange experience of working on unresponsive bodies. And it was also very often at the knife-edge of life and death, an area of medicine that I was never very comfortable with. Physios who specialise in this kind of work are truly remarkable people. And of course that type of work remains as challenging today as it's ever been. Anyway, to lighten the mood once more, let's get back to the stories of yesteryear, the ones that probably should never get out...

There are just two more from my Hull days that still make me laugh today, both involving our boss, John. He 'taught' the unofficial pragmatic and initiative-based approach that has helped me in so many human and equine situations since.

One day, John was treating a patient on the orthopaedic ward who'd had some cartilage removed from his knee. In those days a patient like this would stay in hospital for a week and then be sent home with a pressure bandage and a pair of crutches. But first they had to pass the SLR test (Straight Leg Raise) to prove they had sufficient leg control.

This patient, lying on a bed, seemed to be failing the test. Every time John asked him to lift his leg nothing happened. And John was getting frustrated. So he lifted the man's leg himself, held it a few inches above the bed, got out his cigarette lighter, ignited it – and held it a few inches beneath the man's leg. *"I'm going to count to three and then let go of your leg,"* he explained. *"You'll then need to keep it there, in the air."* This saw an immediate improvement in the man's efforts to comply. Shaking, sweating and swearing the man did manage to keep his leg in the air, and after repeating the test a few time, John declared him fit to go home. Even I can see the point in rules that prevent people lacking

John's skills from taking this kind of risk these days, but you have to remember it was all very different back then.

The final story involves John's deputy, Ken. And Ken was really good at spinal manipulation.

I was struggling with a patient whose neck was really stiff, and I asked Ken if he could help. I'd tried everything I knew and was all too ready to accept. Ken began by telling the patient to lie on his back. Then Ken explained to me and my colleague Sue that we should each take hold of one leg. *"When I tell you, on the count of three, pull."*

We took our positions and waited. *"One, two….three!"* And as we pulled, Ken simultaneously pulled and rotated the man's neck. We heard a loud click and a crack. Then Ken relaxed, let go of the man and cracked his own knuckles – I'll never forget that – and said: *"There we are, problem solved!"* The patient, as white as a sheet, got up slowly from the bed and shuffled away. We never saw him again, so can only presume that the treatment had worked…

I had enjoyed two very happy years at Hull Royal Infirmary. As newly-qualified physios, our inexpert and less than efficient treatment had been nurtured into real medical prowess, and helping people to get better proved hugely satisfying. I also got a big buzz from being part of a multi-disciplinary team where we pulled together to overcome crises and developed tough skins while retaining a real compassion.

But I was beginning to grow hungry for promotion – and for a new location. The travelling was beginning to wear me down a little, and of course the salary remained pitiful. So when a Senior II position became vacant at the local hospital in Goole, I applied. Like Hull, it would be a rotational job across different areas of medicine so I would not be able to specialize. But it was only ten minutes drive from home, and with many of my colleagues also moving on it wasn't too much of a struggle to accept the post when offered it.

What I didn't anticipate as I started the new job was which of the experiences gained at Hull's enormous teaching hospital I would need to transfer and develop further to have a positive impact in the much smaller cottage hospital at Goole. But as always, each experience in life seems to have been put there to prepare me for the next one.

*

Goole is an unusual place, an inland port some miles from the coastline that at its zenith boasted heavy industry and factories. I think some light industry remains today and there is still a working dock with a few ships coming in and out, but the activity is a fraction of what it was even when I was working there in the late-eighties. All that remains of its industrial heyday is a collection of rather grand Victorian houses.

The Goole I got to know, however, was a typical dock town, home to a great many stevedores (dock workers). And a combination of high-risk industrial work and the Wednesday market (an excuse for excessive weekday drinking) meant that once a week we could expect an influx of injuries to sort out. I remember one young chap coming in for treatment completely blathered; he could barely sit on the treatment plinth and almost knocked us out with his breath. I expect today he would be made to go away and sober up first, but we persevered and then left him to catch some much-needed shut-eye, still laid out on the plinth.

Being a cottage hospital, it wasn't really at the cutting edge of surgical work and was unable to offer the same high craftsmanship as at the big city hospitals. So our little hospital catered mainly for simple surgery and some orthopaedic work as well. On the flip side, with none of today's appetite for star and performance ratings for hospitals, we were left in peace to deliver whatever care was possible. But we still, of necessity, had to accept lower standards of outcome expectations; where we might, in Hull, have been able to devise and deliver a comprehensive cure after an accident, in Goole we knew that some patients would be left with some permanent stiffness and weakness. Reflecting on it now, it is clear that this was not at all satisfactory, but we just did the best job we could with what we had.

However, to this young and stubborn Yorkshire woman, any problem was an opportunity. I was by now striding purposefully along my personal and professional journey, and gaining in confidence all the time. To me an inadequate or inefficient medical process was as irritating as petty school rules had been. More than that, it was an excuse for some creative problem solving.

One such problem was simply a shortage of staff. On my very first day in the physio department I was surprised to see the receptionist step out from behind her desk and begin setting up all the equipment. *"What are you doing that for?"* I asked; *"Can't you leave that to the physios?"* *"Oh I've always done it,"* she explained, completely unfazed by having to double up her roles.

In addition to recruitment problems, the department also found it hard to hold onto staff. Goole was not the most exciting of places to work, and physios tended to marry doctors or surgeons who, in their turn, sought more rewarding positions in big teaching hospitals. So we were often understaffed for the number of patients we had to see. And this gave me an idea, one I could easily adapt from my time at Hull. Rather than running ever-lengthening waiting lists we began to group together similar injuries and hold classes for people. This meant that every patient would get from a half to a full hour's group work as well as some one-on-one if they needed it.

Soon we had the department humming like a well-oiled machine with a huge turnover of patients. But there were real health benefits to this as well, not just efficiency gains. My experiences in Hull – both the gym work in the hospital and the rugby club work on the side – had shown me how powerfully people in a group can motivate each other. One-to-one work tends to highlight the individual patient's suffering – and sometimes this is important both to assess the problem and to support the patient. But stick them in groups, and the camaraderie that emerges can achieve so much more. People see other patients better off and worse off, and the instinct to support each other just blossoms.

However, when the physio work is tough, nurturing this camaraderie can require a little hearty 'facilitation' from the staff – and this is where I was in my element. We had classes for hand injuries, shoulders, backs, feet and ankles, knees and hips. And because they were running throughout the day they generated a real momentum and energy. This in turn made it much easier to tighten the screws a little and get faster results. My foot and ankle class became renowned for creating an amiable prisoner-of-war mentality – they knew they were in for a gruelling hour but that didn't stop them on one occasion from applauding me when I turned up to lead the class. And I was soon referred to as the Kampe Kommandant. *"Oh yes, she's bloody good!"* the old hands would say to the new recruits, *"but she'll hurt you!"* One group even brought in some footballs that we used to throw and catch while balancing on tiptoes or on one leg. When the group was discharged at the end of the treatment course, they gave me two of the balls – one inscribed "SAS Training Centre" and the other "Stalag Luft 13". There's something uniquely British about the way a group can rally to face adversity.

Patients weren't the only people to get the tough Katie treatment – I eventually took on the doctors too. I used to get really annoyed by the careless way that our treatments were dictated to us. The physiotherapy referral forms required GPs and consultants to specify the exact physiotherapy treatment to be given – and with little knowledge of what we did, the doctors just put down whichever treatments they had heard of, some of which weren't just unsuitable for the patient in question but downright dangerous. I don't tell the doctors which drugs to use, I thought to myself, so why should they try to tell me my job? However, rather than go head to head with them and disrupt the peaceful running of the little hospital, I decided to reach out with something I knew they would like – an evening of cheese and wine, but served with a generous side-dish of basic physiotherapy education. It was a great success and from then on nearly all referrals stated: "treatment as the physio thinks best".

Of course, being a hospital there were inevitably some sad experiences. One that I always remember was a young man with a family to support who was always in and out of work. And the type of jobs he got seemed to be taking their toll on his back. He came to our department on a regular basis, but we could never identify the source of the problem. In the end we begin to wonder if it was all a ruse or somehow related to his inability to hold down a job. Now, this was all before today's MRI and CAT Scan diagnostics; so, unable to work out what was actually wrong with the guy, our only option was eventually to refer him back to his GP. Finally, however, we did hear of the diagnosis. He'd been suffering from cancer, and within six weeks he was dead.

*

Despite this sad story, I hope I've given an impression of a little cottage hospital that, while being short on resources and cut off from the wider NHS's evolution, nevertheless delivered a good service. However, change did eventually come, and not the kind of change I felt comfortable with. And although I'd been promoted to a Senior I grade, this change was ultimately to encourage me to take the next step in my career. But first, some background.

'Reinventing the wheel' is a phrase that aptly sums up the nonsense that keeps happening in all kinds of public arenas; it occurs whenever the pendulum swings from one tried and tested method to an opposite but equally tried and tested one. It's as if we're incapable of learning and progressing and, instead, have to keep dismantling everything or going backwards. So, the trend in businesses and teamwork today is for bottom-up change – turning to those at the coalface to define the problems, and asking them to help find the solutions too. And it makes good sense, but it's not as new as people think, not at all. In Goole we'd been happily running our own informal equivalent without having to give it a fancy name. We just collaborated regardless of seniority and did what common sense dictated.

However, despite the success of this approach, the day came when we faced the inevitable turn of the cycle of change. Top-down management was making itself felt across the hospital. As a result, people with no clinical or treatment experience were now deciding on our behalf how we could best run the physio department. Their ground-breaking idea was to revert to one-on-one treatment. And of course the obvious consequence happened, as we could have told them had they asked; waiting lists rocketed once more and the gym became like a ghost town. To be honest I have lost touch with current practice in hospitals – but in my experience this pendulum never stops swinging, so you can bet that whatever is considered correct at the moment will all change again pretty soon.

I couldn't go through my entire working life with this periodic disruption, so for me that was my amber light telling me it was nearly time to go it alone and be my own boss. It would cost me a lot of money to set myself up – equipment was not cheap! And I would have to start from scratch with a client list of nil. Nevertheless I was deadly serious about building up my own full-time practice, but it took an additional and very sad trigger to turn the lights from amber to green...

In 1990, my father became seriously ill. He was diagnosed with cancer of the oesophagus and died shortly afterwards. Once I had overcome the initial shock and grief I realized that his death had changed me, but I had to understand how in order to make sense of it. I first noticed that I was beginning to feel frustrated with the patients I saw at hospital; "they only had sprained ankles or pulled shoulders," I grumbled, "whereas my Dad had died from his illness". Of course in time I saw that this was just part of my grief, but it also made me realise that my interest and motivation in the hospital environment had been undermined. And this scared me; I hadn't worked so hard for ten years just to let it all drift away. The way ahead was clear and there was no alternative; I had to seize the reins for myself.

*

I hope these chapters have showed how affectionately I look back on my time in the service. I owe everything I've subsequently been able to do to those early professional years in the NHS. And, without the safety net of a health service and back up of a hospital department, I've had to work hard by myself to show the efficacy of what I do.

But I think going it alone was always on the cards. I needed this challenge of finding and demonstrating the best ways of working with humans and with horses. And I needed freedom from bureaucratic and self-serving management too.

Maybe I also needed this chance to thank my father for the values he'd instilled in me by following in his own entrepreneurial footsteps? Thank goodness he'd taught me not to be afraid of hard work...

CONTAINS:

Part Four – Going it alone
(late 1980s onwards; private practice; early ACPAT and promoting the profession)

Part Five – Equine physiotherapy in detail
(assessments; main problem areas; treatment and case studies)

When my own horses fell or got trapped in drains out hunting, I realized there wasn't a world of difference between their soft tissue injuries and those of the bipeds who we sorted out at hospital. But I think it was probably the experience of taking my physio work beyond the NHS boundaries and into the rugby clubs that really got me thinking: surely I could transfer the techniques to equine care?

Of course I wasn't the first physiotherapist to think this. Like other keen physios I would read our professional journal from cover to cover, and I began to notice some discussion about animal treatment. So when a few physios began advertising in the journal to start a special interest group, I was there, head of the queue. The group was to become ACPAT (Association of Chartered Physiotherapists in Animal Therapy) and for several years I was actively involved (more on this in Chapter 11). And although the group wasn't exclusively aimed at equine work, including working and racing dogs as well, horses made up one of the largest patient groups.

I was also hugely inspired during a trip with Godfrey to South Africa. We'd gone over there to attend a wedding, and I seized the opportunity to seek out an amazing lady, Winks Green, who I had admired from afar. Winks was an incredibly innovative physiotherapist specializing in equines and looking after most of the racehorses in South Africa. She used lunging to help restore fitness to recovering horses and was a great advocate of faradism (electrical muscle stimulation). Her motto was: *"You've got to get right into the injury!"* and her justification was that the horse is a big animal with a dense muscle mass; to improve things post-injury your treatments had to be vigorous in order to mobilize deep structures and scar tissue. She communicated her convictions with such zeal that Godfrey was terrified she might notice some muscle problems in him and insist on treating him.

By this time I had also used physio techniques and equipment myself to treat our beloved hunter, Kasha, when she nearly sliced her leg off in a land drain. So I knew it worked. And in Wressle we had the perfect setting for treating horses – a large yard with stabling for up to twenty horses. All I would need was my electrical equipment plus a few additions like horse walkers, round pens and an arena.

Preparation for going solo had begun while my father was still alive. I'd tried to sell the idea to him but, with his more traditional perspective on animal care, he'd been hard to convince. He'd reckoned that the next thing I'd be trying was putting frogs in the manger. I expect he'd also been concerned that I'd be giving up half of a perfectly good job for possibly nothing. But I think his questioning, perhaps deliberately, spurred me on, and so I stuck to my guns and negotiated a half-time contract at Goole to make space for my own work. I now started putting the word around – I was open for business. And my day would be divided into three parts - the mornings on my rounds treating horses, the afternoons still working at Goole, and then my evenings in a converted bedroom at home where I treated my human clients.

*

When you have spent several years working really hard to acquire the right qualifications to train and work, it is challenging to step into a world devoid of recognized accreditation. But at that time there was no such thing as an equine physiotherapy qualification, so a combination of being Senior I grade in the NHS and an experienced horsewoman had to be good enough. Fortunately our family also had a good reputation locally amongst farmers and the horse world, and they were pretty keen for someone who could treat a core range of typical injuries and conditions. There were even a few vets more than happy to consider my input as a useful option. Nevertheless, when I first set up I hadn't envisaged having to give quite so much time to promoting this new 'thing' called equine physiotherapy (you can read more about how we did this in Chapter 11).

The skepticism from owners right through to very experienced vets was incredible. A little of that remains even today, complicated further by the alternative 'therapists' who want a piece of the action without first slogging to acquire professional skills – the crystal healers and such like. One useful occurrence in the early days was when when a horse was referred with a incorrect diagnosis, and my physio expertise was able to spot this and put it right. This proved a convincing way to persuade people that we really did have something valuable to offer.

However, right at the start I needed some common injuries that I could make visible progress with and that would help to spread the news. And the answer lay with horse racing. This was a useful branch of the equine world as the owners have a lot of money invested in the animals and they need them fit and healthy – in other words, they were eager customers who would, if things went well, be equally eager to spread the word.

Racehorses are not surprisingly prone to falls, and this kept me busy from the start. Using soft tissue manipulation on the horses' backs, sometimes manipulating under sedation, and then prescribing specific exercise, we were able to help send a great many horses back into racing – and remaining upright!

Another type of patient, also common on the racing scene, was the horse that is extremely stiff on the right rein. The problem is evident when you try to lunge the horse in a circle and it will only do squares instead, trying to walk in a straight line, and then stumbling when it has to turn a corner. Nothing has been proven but I think there must be some connection with the way that riders, by tradition, always approach the horse from the left, and also mount and dismount from the left. You see, given that most people are right-handed and may have a tendency to pull more on the right rein, you can begin to see how the horse's muscles can develop unevenly. The horse becomes bent in a way, so when you try to lead them in a circle to the left they resist.

One of the more regular problems that gave me the chance to correct a misdiagnosis as well as treating the horse was laminitis, especially common amongst native ponies bred for the rough terrain. Built for strength and with large bones, these native ponies are slow but phenomenally strong, the diesel engines of the horse world. And with this physique they're generally heavy on their feet, especially if used to pull carts or traps. Their strong forward movement comes from their shoulder muscles, and to facilitate this they tend to have quite a high knee action and heavy footfall. We humans do much the same when we're dragging something heavy behind us. This puts additional stress on the horse's feet with a kind of concussive effect. Throw in the common mistake of letting a horse eat too much protein-rich spring grass and you have a serious problem, laminitis. The laminae inside the wall of the hoof normally acts like a shock absorber for this heavy gait. But with laminitis these become inflamed; and if left untended, the shock of the blood-engorged hoof hitting hard ground is crippling.

The experience of laminitis can be agonizing, like walking barefoot across sharp gravel, so the horse naturally tries to pick up its foot as soon as it touches the ground. However this increases the high-lifting walk, and can create all kinds of muscular problems as the horse distorts its shoulders and back to keep the weight off its feet, hence the complete treatment that a physio can offer.

You can see, I hope, how a good physiotherapist can take a holistic view of a patient, observing both the symptoms and also the behaviours that may relate, something X rays, scans and blood tests alone cannot do. And another good example of this combined technique is in understanding cold-backed horses (where the horse will typically dip away, grunt or otherwise seem unhappy when you saddle them up or do up the girth). With some horses this is just a behavioural habit, but with others it can be a pretty reliable indication of a more serious problem. I remember one case, a rather small hurdler that was very cold-backed. I examined him and could see he was really sore in his back and withers[2]. So we started him on magnetic field therapy and exercise, but he was getting very swollen and hot over his withers. So instead we started some laser treatment to improve circulation, and things quickly and literally came to a head. Very soon it was like Vesuvius erupting! It transpired he had fistulous withers, probably caused by an ill-fitting saddle, and having got the circulation going again the fistula just came to the boil. We wouldn't normally choose electrical treatment where an infection is present, but in this case it helped give us the early diagnosis and speed up the cure. All we had to do then was clean up the wound, give the horse some antibiotics and use the laser to heal the floor of the wound.

Of course, with a horse comes an owner; and even with good assessment and examination procedures, I soon learned how important it can be to extract vital information from the owner. Without this I couldn't always work out exactly what was wrong and how to put it right. Not all owners, however, were very forthcoming.

One such case was a high-quality eventer who came to me with a reported shoulder problem – I was told he had soreness in the shoulder and in the brachiocephalicus[3] on the near side. This was soothed with treatment – but then kept coming back. I realised that the original diagnosis, and possibly the supporting information, cannot have been entirely accurate. I looked for signs of swelling or heat in the leg but couldn't find anything. So in the end I deduced that the horse must have had some kind of fall or slip and, sensibly enough, I asked if the owner could verify this. *"No! Absolutely not. How dare you suggest that!"* Well, that left

[2] The ridge between the shoulder blades of an animal
[3] Long, flat muscle that extends from intersection claviuclaris between brachium and the head and neck

me with no option other than to refer the horse back to the vet. There, as he was a bit upright in his pasterns[4], they decided to do a scan – and they found a DDFT[5] lesion, the tell-tale sign of an accident. So now he could at last get the right treatment and rest and then resume his career.

Sometimes it is not an accident that the owner is ashamed of but the relationship with their horse. On occasions, once I start to treat a horse for a physical condition, the owner opens up a little and begins telling me of difficulties they are experiencing. And it is very rewarding to be able to help matters a little. Every horse has its own personality, and horses and people can clash. Some horses by nature are easy-going, 'push-button' animals obedient and eager to please. Others however may be more feisty, and if challenged by their owner they will challenge back, for example by bucking. It's their way of saying: "I don't like that; don't do it to me!" And horses, like dogs, can show self-awareness; I'm always incredulous of people who dress their horse up in flashy Christmas gear to impress the owner's friends – and then wonder why the horse bucks them off.

Some behavioural problems are not really problems at all, just understandable traits that are overlooked by blasé owners. For example it's easy for a horse to be spooked by a dark, windy lane; and it's not unsurprising for it to respond by bucking and galloping off. The insensitive owner brays the horse indignantly when she catches up, which sadly just reinforces the negative experience and increases the chance of it happening again.

It would be easier if people didn't attach stigma to behavioural problems; much better to be up front and honest about it. But some owners are cautious or coy and initially don't tell me about the problem (or are simply in denial about it). For me, it is doubly satisfying to diagnose and treat both a physical injury and the

---

[4] the part between the fetlock and the hoof
[5] deep digital flexor tendon (between the horse's elbow and knee)

relationship or behavioural issue that ultimately led to the incident. But I do need to have that frank conversation with the owner, especially if I end up recommending some tough behavioural rehabilitation work. Of course, for those owners who simply want to enjoy their horse for pleasure and relaxation, challenging rehab work can simply be too big an undertaking. The best thing for them then is to admit dignified defeat and part with their horse before things deteriorate further. It's no different to human relationships really – clashes can erupt, and some can be resolved while others just can't.

Another source of behavioural work came from riggy horses[6]. Nowadays you only get a riggy gelding when a vet has been a bit jumpy and not done the cleanest of jobs, but there was a time when they were left like this deliberately to give the gelding a nice neck and topline. And some of these horses are fine – no behavioural problems at all. But for others it can leave them with weird and quirky traits. Put a riggy boy with a mare in season and anything might happen. Godfrey has one at the moment – Sydney – and he put him in the field with a mare; Sydney just clung to her, gave a kind of squeal and then peed. But you have to be wary of rehab work. Some can be really aggressive and unpredictable; others are fine except for a tendency to try to mate with anything in their field...

Finally, as in any medical field, there are sad cases, treatment that doesn't go well and horses that have to be destroyed. When I first worked for myself, this happened most when I was only approached as the last resort, the last glimmer of hope, before the inevitable euthanasia. But sometimes bad things just happen – it's just part of life.

There was a lovely old show jumper whose joints had lost their shock absorption capability. We were able to improve his back

---

[6] Following castration a small part of the epidymis is left behind and continues to produce hormones

and neck for a few days at a time but then his stride would shorten again. Sadly there was nothing to be done. Latterly I was able to experience this for myself when my hips finally gave up. I used to run a lot and suddenly I lost my athletic stride and I could actually hear my feet just slapping on the ground. I know how that poor horse must have felt.

Another sad one was a yearling colt who had been mucking about with his mates. He'd reared up and got his near foreleg over the back of another horse which then pulled away, leaving him with an avulsion injury that resulted in a brachial plexus[7] lesion. This left him without any fetlock, knee or elbow extension. We eased things a little with muscle stimulation but, being only a yearling, his other front leg wasn't strong enough to cope with the additional pressure it was getting. I worked with a splinting company but whatever we tried caused pressure sores. In the end the inevitable had to happen.

And a final example shows how pointless these sad cases can be - a horse that got a puncture wound from a kick and developed an infection. It wasn't this that did him in but the fact he had flexed his leg so much in response to the pain that it had contracted his hamstrings too much for us to stretch them out again. You wouldn't believe just how depressing some of these cases can be. And of course you try to remain positive for the sake of the owner, especially if the horse has already done the circuit of vets and other specialists and their only hope now is for the physio to perform a miracle. But nothing can take away the disappointment and anger when a fine animal has to be destroyed because of one untreatable injury.

---

[7] the network of nerves that conducts signals from the spinal cord to the shoulder and limb

No responsible owner would let anyone near their animal unless they knew they could be trusted. And nowadays when I'm working on a horse, the owner usually has some understanding already of what I'm trying to do. Back in the late 1980s, however, there were a lot of owners, plenty of riding schools and even a few vets who had very little idea of equine physiotherapy. So first we had to answer the question above by promoting our work. And that was almost a full-time job in itself.

The launch of ACPAT – the Association of Chartered Physiotherapists in Animal Therapy –in 1985 kicked off the process as the official face for what had been growing embryonically for some time. And one of the first achievements of the organization was to effect an amendment to the Royal College of Veterinary Surgeon's (RCVS) constitution.

Prior to ACPAT's amendment, this constitution stated that only a member of the RCVS could diagnose and treat an animal; our amendment changed this to include physiotherapy treatment on referral from a vet who had made the diagnosis, and today all ACPAT therapists must be members of the Chartered Society of Physiotherapists (MCSP[8]). This was a big step; it effectively opened up a new branch of multi-disciplinary working in the veterinary field. However, compared to my hospital work, where we were by now being regarded as equal clinical team members able to help diagnose and select our own treatments, this felt like going backwards. We were definitely at the end of the veterinary care food chain but we had to start somewhere.

At the start ACPAT was a very small organization headed by Mary Bromiley (who held the twin post of President and

---

[8] Member of the Chartered Society of Physiotherapists

Chairwoman). The idea was to develop treatment for a wide range of animals including some exotica, but very soon a particular focus developed on working animals - horses and dogs – whose owners needed them to be back up and running as quickly as possible. Mary lived in Marlborough and ran a rehabilitation yard for racehorses. Being well connected with the racing world and the Jockey Club she got good access to the right people high up – as with anything, who you know can make all the difference.

These were very exciting times for us, but there was so much missionary work to do. And this took the twin form of external promotion – to the vets whose referrals we would rely on and to the owners who needed to see what we could do – and internal peer support. We were all experienced and professionally accredited physios, but we still needed to share our emerging animal expertise amongst ourselves and learn from each other.

So what we really needed was some efficient organizational structure and good admin – all the unglamorous stuff that no one enjoys! To make matters worse, the numerous special interest physio groups that exist today (sports, medicine, neurology, etc) were thin on the ground, so we couldn't simply adopt their frameworks. We knew we had a steep hill to climb if we were to build on our early momentum to become a permanently established part of the treatment package available to horses and other animals.

And so, full of enthusiasm as ever, I volunteered and got stuck in.

By 1988 I had joined the ACPAT committee and took an immediate interest in two particular lines of work – the newsletter and the conferences. The newsletter was a simple quarterly journal to help spread the word and encourage new ACPAT members. There was a basic membership for people with a passing interest - *"Oh that looks a bit of fun..."* - and this membership would fluctuate. But there was another level for people who worked professionally with horses and, by including liability insurance in the package, it attracted more serious members who wanted to develop their equine practice.

I suppose my main input, however, was in the courses and conferences that we ran all over the country. In the early days members were invited to two annual seminars (spring and autumn), one-day events when we would meet up at someone's stables or riding school. There would be talks from physios on their equine work, and sometimes we'd get vets to come and speak on anatomy and other topics. Eventually this grew into two-day conferences with an equal focus on horses and other animals, and these were open to non-members too. And of course somewhere in there we'd tuck the AGM, as well as some kind of evening social event.

We became really good at this PR work – and we knew how to attract some amazing speakers using generous fees and warm hospitality. I felt it a privilege to represent the pioneering ACPAT in places as far afield as Edinburgh, Glasgow, Liverpool, London and Newmarket. And because innovation attracts innovation, I was lucky to meet some inspiring and pioneering vets too. But there was still that hands-on part of me that was itching to do more than just organize events and host speakers. So it wasn't long before I found myself venturing into physiotherapy demonstrations.

They always say never to go on the stage with children or animals; but taking a pantomime horse with me wasn't an option. And in any case, how can you possibly demonstrate horse physiotherapy without a horse? Of course, just like people, horses are vulnerable to stage fright, leading to the inevitable 'accident' – but that just helps everybody to relax, and as my demonstrations were always in riding clubs or agricultural colleges, they were used to manure!

My ACPAT demos took me to colleges like Myerscough and Moreton Morrell where the audiences were keen and interested to learn. And I found I loved being up there in front of them with a horse, showing real live anatomy and movement. It's different to riding and jumping at a show; here you're not competing but you still get to be the star attraction (well, after the horse of course) – and it always felt like a stage show; so perhaps, in a way, I finally got the performance opportunity that the choirmaster at Queen Margaret's had so roughly denied me?

Unfortunately not all our Public Relations targets were so enthusiastic. Vets could be very tricky. Some were simply skeptical of what we could bring to the table, but others, I think, felt professionally threatened; instead of regarding us as useful specialists to have on their informal team, they saw us as trying to steal part of their own territory. Yet others were just greedy and saw us as competition for their revenue.

Interestingly I got a glimpse of where this mentality might first set in when I was lecturing at the University of Cambridge Veterinary College. It was a prestigious invitation, although the initial connection had been an unusual one. Godfrey kept popping off to Cambridge in the '90s to do some more professional exams and he used to meet up there with his goddaughter who was a student. After one particularly boozy evening of which he had no memory, he woke the next morning to discover that he had agreed to sponsor the university's Ladies' Rugby team. It then transpired that a few members of the team were studying veterinary science, and thus the connection was made.

So there I was, giving a well-prepared and in-depth lecture to what I presumed was the cream of veterinary students. And when it came to the time for questions, one hand shot up. I braced myself for some sharp intellectual drilling. *"I don't understand how it all works,"* the student said; *"who gets the fee, you or us?"* I guess I had just expected them to be a little more vocational in their attitude. After all there are easier ways to make money than by being a vet!

As my own work developed, however, I was lucky. I soon developed a strong reputation with my local vet practices and was able to work on a blank referral basis; they were happy to send their patients to me, knowing that I could confirm or question their diagnosis, and that if I was in any doubt about anything I'd get back to them immediately. They could see for themselves how the physiotherapy could help them and didn't need further convincing. And I like to think that some of our early ACPAT lectures and demonstrations had helped to create this collegial atmosphere.

*

So, helping to get ACPAT off the ground was an incredibly busy task but I wouldn't have missed it for the world. Being in at the start of something is so much more exciting, even if your head frequently aches from being banged against so many brick walls. And my business was going really well too. But for me the real reward was still all about the hands-on work – as I'll now explain...

I readily admit that my academic career was pretty middle of the road. So you won't be surprised to hear that I had never imagined I'd ever become any kind of teacher. However, working on behalf of ACPAT helped to develop my presentation and lecturing skills (and confidence), and soon I began to be invited to speak and teach on my own merits.

Riding clubs were growing keen to find out more, especially with the volume of small accidents and injuries that come with the job. And I found I was able to combine the remedial physio part of my talks with practical tips and exercises to keep horse and ponies healthy – a kind of proactive injury prevention. Vets invited me too. The more go-ahead practices had already begun to put on special interest events to impress and retain their clients, and my topic was an obvious candidate for these.

A talk that I shall never forget, however, was my one and only dip into the world of complementary health for animals. Clearly my new-age audience shared my interest in resolving problems and treating injuries, but I don't think our methods had much in common. I stuck to my core routine, covering the physiology, the nature of injuries and the range of physiotherapeutic interventions – but I faced an unwelcoming sea of rather blank faces. They, it seemed, favoured crystal healing, reiki and even some spiritualist techniques. I don't think I made much of an impression. I've no problem with people following their own chosen paths, but I don't think these treatments have much to offer the athletic horse. And from a business perspective, it was a useful reminder to me to know and grow my own market!

I also took a part-time role teaching HND and degree-level equine students at Bishop Burton College in Yorkshire. I loved this immensely, and it allowed me to indulge in my no-nonsense approach too; I demanded complete attention from my students.

I'm not sure if today's colleges encourage this style, but it worked for me. If there was any disturbance or lack of concentration I would stop in my tracks and wait for silence; then I'd deliver the standard lines – 1) *"You're paying a vast amount of money for me to stand here and teach you,"* and 2) *"If you're not interested, you can leave the room immediately."* To be honest I rarely had to resort to this; they were an enthusiastic crowd (such a contrast to the Cambridge students) and always had loads of excellent questions to ask – keeping me on my toes!

*

So by now, with my own equine practice firmly established and my name getting known on the lecture circuit as well, things were going pretty well. But it wasn't all about horses; I was still running my human practice in my physio studio at Wressle. By now the mania for keep-fit and marathon running had never been hotter and this kept me extremely busy. People eager to experience the pleasures and highs of running long distances often lacked adequate training – although sometimes Mother Nature had simply not given them the best mechanical assets to match their enthusiasm.

So I'd be working with knock knees, bow legs and flat feet, but I always found ways to help them get the most from what they had by going beyond just the physical assessment. I would talk about the type of shoes, the part of the road or camber to use, and about their general running technique. True to form, I could be quite ruthless if I had to; after all, these people were paying for my help, so I didn't hold back with the criticism where it mattered. And some clients were so enthusiastic but then so bad at keeping up with their exercises that I had to play a serious tough cop, saying I'd sack them if they didn't pull their socks up. *"My reputation is everything – and you're an advertisement for it. You won't let me down!"* And it always worked. I was known for being expensive but extremely good.

And on the subject of my fee, I've included a little anecdote at the end of this chapter that I'd love to share with you. It's as much about how, when you're working really hard, you can easily overlook the fact that you've achieved something impressive. You just keep your head down and keep on working. Fortunately I had my fan-base, Godfrey, and he wasn't going to let this pass me by completely.

*

I was by now very aware of how it felt to be doing well. But it wasn't the business success that I relished so much as the sheer enjoyment and reward of the physiotherapy work itself. And a significant part of this was the need to use initiative. I look back to the '80s and '90s and am staggered to remember just how few books we had to learn from, in fact how little was known then and how much we had to pioneer. Physiotherapists in the early days certainly needed to be enthusiastic, innovative and determined, drawing on the core guidelines inherent in McKenzie exercises, Maitland manipulation and PNF[9] techniques. I suppose I'm one of those people who are always happiest carving their own way rather than simply following a pre-determined course – so it had suited me very well.

But the real buzz was, and remains, the process of helping a person or a horse feel better. My own style of work – being very hands-on – means I'm really in touch with how the patient is experiencing it; and it can be hard work for them! Manual therapy, whether massage, soft tissue mobilization or manipulation, can be extremely uncomfortable or even painful when you have an acute or chronic problem as the muscles tend to hold you rigid and set like concrete. So my task is to pummel, pull and push until the muscle regains some elasticity.

---

[9] proprioceptive neuromuscular facilitation

Patients talk of feeling like they've been run over by a steam roller, but once the bruising wears off and mobility returns, the relief and confidence on the patient's face says it all. I meanwhile am suffering for my efforts – my arms, fingers, wrists and elbows feel ready to drop off. But the patient, both human and equine, will often feel suddenly sleepy after treatment – stretching a little, yawning and getting comfortable as their muscles relax. And seeing that is a satisfaction that has never diminished at all in all the years I've been doing this.

Before the anecdote I promised you earlier, I want to visit a different perspective to this reflection on the trappings of success with something slightly different, the other side of the coin I suppose, a type of failure.

Godfrey and I have no children, but it's not for want of trying. By the mid 1990s, with nothing happening in that department, we decided to try IVF. Three attempts and three non-survivor implanted embryos later and I was feeling pretty desperate. So we decided to consider egg donation. And I am convinced that what happened next was fate playing its cunning hand…

We get an appointment to discuss the process in Nottingham and drive down there, arriving slightly late. So I rush into the waiting room while Godfrey parks the car. I'm sitting there flicking through a magazine without taking in any of the words and I look up. My eyes meet those of a girl sitting opposite, only for a split second but long enough for me to recognize her. "*I know you,*" I think to myself; "*I was at school with you, and bumped into you at a reunion; you've been married, you had kids, then you divorced.*" But when she comes over to chat, I keep these thoughts to myself.

She asks what I'm doing there so I tell her – and guess what, she's there to donate her eggs. At that moment Godfrey finally arrives, just in time as the consulting room door opens and our names are called. As I walk through it is like a light switch flicking in my mind; I don't want *her* eggs, I realize; and in fact I don't want to be playing with nature at all, full stop.

Of course it wasn't that simple, not really. Afterwards I was in pieces and I felt that I had failed. So I did my best to rally round and make sense of it all. Family had always been a central part of my life, and now, since it was clear that I couldn't build my own, I had no alternative but to fill the gap by achieving even more with my work and my horses. That was how I tried to make sense of it. And I sometimes wonder if fate had intervened too, given the troublesome period that followed.

It began with my mother's health deteriorating, causing breathing problems and a lot of hospitalization. Then I hit the menopause ahead of time in my early forties. At the same time my hands developed carpal tunnel syndrome – and as a hands-on physio it was important to have this properly rectified with surgery. And I was still showing horses but it was becoming a real nuisance and interfering with my support for Godfrey's hobbies. And finally my own beloved hobby, hunting, was about to banned.

To bring a young child into all of that might have been one thing too many for our marriage, especially as politics was about to take up residence in our household. But am I still sad not to have children? I daren't really think about it.

And here, at last, is that anecdote…

Yorkshire values - you are what you drive.

I am not, and never have been, interested in superficial appearances. When I choose my clothes for the day, they're matched to whatever tasks lie ahead. First thing in the morning there are much more urgent things to sort out – dogs to walk, horses to turn out, husbands to chivvy – so with me, like it or not, you get a practical wardrobe governed by the prevailing weather, and that's it.

But there's a professional reason for this too. Working with nervous patients is all about reassurance; you may be about to do some undignified and intrusive things to them and you need them to have confidence in you. They want to see you dressed for the task in hand, looking competent, tidy and clean and clearly focused on them, not on your catwalk score for the day.

So what's all this got to do with driving?

Living remotely in the flat expanse of the Vale of York, a car is a necessity. But I've always enjoyed the cars I've owned. I was so proud of my first car, a Mini Metro, (the trend-setter when hatchbacks were still a novelty). Ok, so it was dressed in British Leyland's signature sh*t-brown paintwork and beige nylon upholstery, but it was mine and I loved it. Whizzing between Wressle and Hull I felt Queen of the Road. And did it whizz! On a trip to the Lake District I remember briefly touching the magic ton…

However, the bare fact is that people often judge you on what you drive. And amongst the farming and equestrian communities, the benchmarks are subtle. Aim too high and they'll think you're going to rip them off; rattle around in a rusty bone-shaker and you're deemed to be unreliable and on the way out of business.

My own cars have always been utilitarian workhorses first, and reliable and adequately comfortable transport second – never fashion statements. And this seemed to go down well with my clients and customers – especially the monosyllabic Yorkshire farmers so skillfully portrayed by James Herriott and still in evidence to this day. Their reputation, however, for being cheapskates or bargain hunters is undeserved. I prefer to think of them as shrewd judges of value. Mean? Sometimes. Penny-pinching? Occasionally. But cheapskates? Definitely not. They simply live according to a very sound principle; you should not have to pay a penny more for anything than it is actually worth.

So, when I had left the NHS and was working solo, my car at the time, a well-kept duck-egg blue Morris Minor Traveller, hit just the right neutral tone. Devoid of snobbery, it communicated nothing about my wealth, or lack of. And the Morris was British through and through, basic but characterful, a sensible car, beloved of health visitors up and down the country. It invited trust – just what I needed when dealing with people who still saw me as just a cheaper alternative to t' vit'nary.

However, behind every great woman lurks a man with ambition, and while my modest transport suited me to the ground, Godfrey had other ideas. This is the same Godfrey who nowadays smooches around the countryside in a classy Jaguar sports. Godfrey likes quality cars. So it was inevitable I suppose that one day he would tire of seeing me driving 'vans with back seats'.

Don't misunderstand him; he wasn't trying to tart up his Yorkshire wife. Even though he still likes to surprise me with extravagant new frocks (for me, not for him), he respects the integrity of my usual work attire. But once he gets an idea, that's it. So he decided one day that my professional standing needed more visibility – I'd earned it apparently. And his solution? A brand new Mercedes C-Class Estate, my first seriously smart and sophisticated vehicle.

Of course I was delighted – it was a super looking machine, oozing quality and wonderfully comfortable too. But was it really me? And how would it go down with my least amenable clients, the kind of people who tried to wriggle out of paying for anything, especially for what they still regarded as 'new-fangled mumbo jumbo'? I was about to find out...

My first visit in the new car is to a large and untidy livery yard in West Yorkshire. The owner is an old-fashioned farmer who uses a billy band instead of a belt to hold up his baggy and grubby trousers. His creased and tanned face clearly hasn't felt a close shave for decades. He watches as I carefully steer my executive ride through narrow gates and around the larger of the potholes in the main yard.

"Bludy 'ell lass! What the 'ell yer chargin' these days?"

A good Yorkshire statement – no subtlety, straight to the point. He is ungallant too, watching but offering no help as I step elegantly from the car and land straight in a large shitty puddle. So I respond in an equally brusque fashion.

"That's right Jim, I make good money. And you know why? Success and results; that's what you're paying for!"

I'm not always so quick with the sharp comeback, but Godfrey has coached me well. And it has certainly shut Jim up as he stomps off heavily, leading me towards the stables.

Looking back on this now, I remember thinking it was ok. I knew Jim well, and while he'd moan about it to his mates down the pub, I could tell that he was impressed, both by the car and by my quick retort. You see, Yorkshire people may not like dishing out their money, but they certainly do understand the value of things. You just have to explain it in the right way – the blunt way.

There is actually more to this story – but I'll keep it brief. My prestigious executive car proved to be less than we'd hoped; within a few months the tailgate began rotting right through. Leaving aside the detrimental impact this had on my hard-earned status symbol, to Godfrey it was simply unacceptable. However the garage, like they do, saw things less urgently than he did and unwisely tried to fob him off with stories of delayed parts and so on. This was met with a typical Godfrey response: *"Either you mend or replace this car right now, or I shall park in front of your garage every day with a large notice pointing to the rotting bodywork and warn people not to buy a Mercedes from you. The choice is yours."* And I know Godfrey; he would have done exactly that, and rather enjoyed it I expect.

A word about this section of the book...

I was in two minds about whether to include a detailed explanation of the actual hands-on equine work, but I have been told that many readers will enjoy dipping into this. So I've pulled together some case studies and background information that reflect the three core elements of the job – assessment, treatment and rehabilitation. However, with thousands of sets of case notes safely stored in filing cabinets, choosing ones that are sufficiently detailed without being impossible to read was not easy; I hope I've made the right selection.

Now, if the idea of this section doesn't appeal, feel free to jump to Section 3 of the book where you'll be taken to the worlds of showing and selling horses, hunting, sidesaddle riding – and Godfrey. But if you have the stamina, stick with it – you may just find it rather interesting!

"So tell me, where does it hurt?"

And therein lies the problem; horses can't tell you. But this is also what makes the work so fascinating.

Working therapeutically with animals requires infinite skill – in all it took me three years of hard training, eight years of NHS experiential work and another sixteen years since then to learn everything I've learned. And as I cannot possibly share all of that here, what I can do in the first chapter of this section is to give you a good idea of how I assess a horse – how I discover what it might tell me, if only it could.

It will be a long read but I hope it will be interesting and give a good insight into what I'm looking for and expecting to treat; and if you find either yourself or your horse at a physio consultation, you will have a better understanding of what might be going on. It goes without saying that this chapter isn't a DIY guide – these may appear simple techniques but they do require considerable expertise if you are to avoid a misdiagnosis and then make things worse!

I think, unless you have veterinary experience, it is best to approach the following three chapters as informative, not educational. They may give you a better hunch about when your own horse is in trouble, but you should still always consult the professionals first; home-remedies rarely work and can make things much worse for your horse.

Having said that, if you do have a injured horse it may well require extensive rehabilitation and exercise therapy for maximum recovery, and that will definitely involve you directly under your vet's or physio's guidance. So I talk about this as well. As with humans, mechanical injuries can take a long, long time to be fully treated, and the process is one of patient and painstaking rehab. If you find yourself facing a long convalescent period with your horse, your vet or physio will make sure you fully understand what you are to do and why; I hope my comments on the topic will give you the confidence to take on this important work.

Finally, bear in mind that some of my work harks back to the pioneering years in the profession when, in the absence of modern technology, we had to rely so much more on our hands-on expertise. Today, if your horse has an accident, there are some amazing machines and medical devices that can really speed up treatment and recovery. Just one example is the range of modern dressings that help to heal a wound much faster, before it really breaks down – something I didn't get to use for many years. But just remember that if things progress slower than you'd hoped, or the final stage of healing seems unattainable, it may be that we physios can identify the missing piece of the jigsaw.

Given my appetite for diagnostic work, you won't be surprised that my assessment process is pretty thorough. It's obvious that this initial examination and conversation with the patient or the owner is crucial to whatever treatment is chosen, but believe me, there are plenty of medical consultations that don't seek the same degree of information at the outset. I talked recently to a newly-retired GP who was horrified to read a medical journal article talking of GPs doing away altogether with face to face examinations. A computer and a skype account are, apparently, all that's required...

But to me, for humans and horses alike, there are some great clues to be found through close-up observation – everything from the posture, the look in the eye, the way the patient moves and positions himself in the room or the stable, the visible condition (skin, hair, coat, etc). I actually crossed swords with a group of NHS physios at a conference when I tried to explain how I assess horses using these clues. They thought I was mad, but in my opinion if they don't do the same with their human patients, then they're not doing a very good job. They're like the GP who spends the first few precious minutes of a brief consultation paying attention to computer notes instead of you; it's a wasted diagnostic opportunity. Of course computers and the internet have created another problem, the over-informed patient. My former physio tutor, Alex Fuller, was complaining recently about how everyone now hankers after a 'recipe book' of ailments and treatments, brainwashed by their experience of the internet into expecting instant answers to everything. The trouble is that people – and animals – are not like computers; each individual reacts differently and so each treatment and technique must be adapted to each patient.

With both horses and humans, the initial assessment is like a detective story – you find out what happened, when it happened, where, how - and my job is to take these jigsaw pieces and begin to assemble the picture. My assessments will appear rather old-fashioned to some younger physiotherapists, but I find they help minimize the risk of my missing a crucial clue. In fact, I can safely say that with this method I never miss anything. It even reveals enough for me to be able to sense when an owner is being economical with some useful background facts.

Here's a simple example – and it's good old laminitis once more! Just the other day I visited a client. She couldn't pin down what was wrong with her horse but told me five things about it: 1) she assured me it was in better condition than it had ever been (a touch defensive I wondered?); 2) it had a good appetite and was enjoying the lush grass; 3) it was usually full of energy and galloping around a lot, but 4) it seemed recently to have become a bit fretful; and 5) it was lying down a lot. The last two pieces of information somewhat contradicted the first, but I had a good hunch straightaway. And following my usual assessment process (detailed below) I ascertained two crucial indicators to bear out my hunch: 1) in movement he was very pottery in the front end, wanting to take the weight off his front feet; 2) his shoulder muscles and pectorals were extremely tight on both sides and clearly very painful. I knew exactly what it was, and contacted the vet who was then able to prescribe deep shavings in the stable, an immobilized horse and a reduced diet. The horse recovered.

So, here's my assessment process exactly as I will normally conduct it, and starting with my kit.

Assessment kit

My basic kit simply comprises a clipboard, a pre-formatted A5 assessment sheet, a reliable pen, and a milk crate (more on this shortly). It also includes the most important items, my eyes and hands. At this stage all of the work is observation and history-taking, building up layers of information, each of which can reveal vital information. And the history begins with the obvious – the horse's date of birth. If the horse is only four or five, it may be too inexperienced and underdeveloped for the way it's been ridden;

equally a much older horse could well be suffering wear and tear of the joints. I also consider the breed of horse and the job it does. A 'happy hacker's' horse probably only goes out once or twice a week and may not be very fit and therefore is susceptible to muscle pulls, while a three-day eventer or show jumper can suffer the same injuries and strains as a champion human athlete. These are all useful pointers or ways to confirm subsequent findings.

The assessment - pre-examination

Sometimes, as in the laminitis example above, I can diagnose a simple problem very easily from talking to the owner and just a brief examination. But at its fullest my assessment incudes the horse's initial presentation, its physical symmetry and its movement; then I test reflexes, and explore the muscles with palpation[10]; and finally I may measure swelling in affected joints and test for excessive heat as well.

But before any of this it's sometimes really helpful just to find out more about the owner's experience of the horse. It can be revealing to ask, for example, if the horse normally enjoys rolling but not recently, or is only going down on one side. The same goes for how the horse behaves when being saddled or when the girth is tightened. And when the owner mounts the horse does it raise its back, or perhaps move as if to sit down? And what about how it is to ride - does it seem to have a preferred diagonal (often the result of the rider not sitting square and evenly balanced)? And, when cantering, are all the legs working smoothly in the right order, or is it a bit like riding a bicycle with a flat tyre?

There are still more questions to put before I actually need to meet the horse. I need to ask about its the current symptoms (*when did you first notice them? How often do they show?*). I want to know about its medical history, any old injuries, surgery, a previous

---

[10] Using the hands to examine the body

instance of the current problem and so on. For example, an issue with a right limb might actually arise from overcompensating after an old injury to the corresponding left limb. So again, by methodically playing detective I can elicit potentially useful information before even beginning my examination. Of course, some owners can be economical with the truth, especially if their carelessness has caused the problem, but over the years I've become better at spotting this in our initial conversation.

And I'm still not quite ready to examine the horse – I first need to note down any medication currently prescribed and look at any X-rays the vet might already have taken. And I usually get the owner to repeat what the vet will already have told me, just to make sure we don't all end up confused and contradicting each other. I also take care to help the owner understand that although their horse is 'the best horse in the world' (or so they think) I will of necessity be very blunt in the way I describe it – and I tell them not to be offended!

Now, at last, I'm ready to start the examination. And it begins with simple observation.

The assessment - examination

You can learn a lot from the way the horse presents in the stable – is it up front, curious and alert? Does it linger at the back in the shadows? Does it seem happy? And do its ears prick up when it sees its owner approaching? If I've been called on a more behavioural than medical mission, it's really useful also to observe the horse's attitude towards the owner; if it knocks him/her about a bit it clearly doesn't have much respect. Or perhaps I may notice that the owner is overhandling the animal.

Symmetry

I then observe more closely to assess the horse's symmetry. This is about the general shape of the horse and the way it holds itself, and obviously it differs from breed to breed. But a healthy animal, as with a human, should have a basic symmetry between left and right. So I get the owner to stand the horse square while I observe first from one side and then the other; then from the front and finally the back (and that's where the milk crate comes in – standing on it gives me a better view along the back). If I notice any asymmetry I make a note but also bear in mind it might just be a signpost towards the real problem area; for example, really bad feet could mean a resulting problem with the shoulders and knees.

Movement

And now the movement observation begins. I always work my way through the same steps and in this order: I want to see the horse walking, then trotting; I want to see it walking in tight circles, to observe its ability to turn its head and neck; and I want to see how well it walks backwards. Let me just say a little about each of these.

Walking: I need to see the horse walking away from me and back to me, in a straight line, and also watch from both sides as it is led past me. I'm looking for a nice comfortable length of stride with relaxed and elastic movement rather than stiff wooden plodding. I also like to see what happens when it's on the turn as this can reveal a weakness in its feet or joints. I'm watching to see if the feet fall nice and straight when turning or land on the inner or outer border. Posture when walking can be a good give-away of a problem. A tense walk with a very upright head and short mincing steps tell me a lot about what is happening in the back muscles.

Trotting: Because it is a tauter movement (compare your own slow, relaxed stroll with a gentle running gait) a limp or other weakness can show more clearly in a trotting horse. As well as watching the footfall and the nod of the head, I can more easily see whether the horse is moving crookedly or straight. If a horse is tight in its back it will curve slightly when trotting and you can then see one buttock or hip being held higher than the other. You can also notice how well aligned or not the front and rear feet are in a trot. The tail being held to one side can be a good indication of a sore back (the tail favouring the side with the stronger muscle), but you need to consider the breed – some such as arabs and welsh types have a natural tendency to lift and turn the tail over itself.

Circles: This is one test that definitely benefits from a skilled owner or assistant who can stand still by the horse's shoulder while leading it round in tight circles in both directions. You're effectively trying to get the horse to bend itself closely around the handler, almost walking on the spot, and the technique involves pulling the head inwards with a lead rein while pushing its rear quarters away at the same time. An inexperienced handler can easily end up being stood on. But when you get it right, the horse is then taking really tiny steps and you can observe how the back is bending and how well the horse is crossing its hind legs to facilitate the tight turn. A horse with tight hips, hocks or stifles won't want to bring the inside leg forward and across because it will hurt. Alternatively, the horse might willingly put its weight on the leg that has to do this to relieve pain in the other leg. And of course, if it has a stiff or painful neck, it won't want to turn into the tight circle at all.

Walking backwards: If you've ever had a limp you may well have walked by taking a larger step with the bad leg, and then a shorter one to quickly restore balance with the good one; that way you also cover ground faster. With horses you can spot this indication easily when they walk backwards. You gently push the horse from the front and, if healthy, it will keep in a straight line with its legs aligned and the head slightly dropped, and walk with a supple and soft movement. But the horse with a problem will take the same alternating long and short strides as we do, and usually end up veering off course, a bit like rowing a boat and working one oar much more than the other. If it has a tight back, the horse will hold its head up. And with a bad back, this will hurt and the horse will begin to resist.

There's one last movement test – the carrot stretches. I want to see how well the horse can turn and lower its head when standing still. And few horses can resist a juicy carrot. You position the horse alongside a wall and with his bottom in the corner so that he is as square as possible and can't shuffle away. Then using the carrot as lure, you get him to turn his head to his elbow, maybe a little further towards his hind leg. If he has any stiffness he'll try to turn his body to reach the carrot. You also take the carrot between his front legs to see how well he can drop his head – to his chest, his knees and then his fetlocks. If he has stiffness he may try to compensate by walking backwards

So, by now I will have made comprehensive notes on the horse's movement and posture and any obvious difficulties. It's time to look at the reflex systems. And can I stress here the importance of not trying this yourself? You can easily upset and hurt your horse!

Reflexes

With reflex testing I'm trying to elicit responses in the ventral and dorsal reflexes and also monitor how quickly it recovers. A fit horse, unhampered by stiff or painful muscles, will show a normal reflex response and then return quickly and smoothly to its previous posture.

The problem is that each horse, as well as each breed, has different reflex responses – there's no hard and fast standard to measure against. Also, this process can be irritating to a horse so I have to be sensitive to how it reacts if I am to interpret what I see accurately. But what I'm looking for is a satisfactory normal response to a reflex trigger; anything else can indicate soreness and stiffness.

If you stroke a horse really quickly and briskly down its back muscle, from where the saddle sits and along its spine, you should see the horse dip its back and flex sideways. The speed of this response depends on the breed; a thoroughbred's response will be quite fast while that of a cobby type of heavy horse is slower. If the back is sore you'll see one of two things; the horse might almost drop to the floor in surprise and discomfort (and this is why it is so important to adjust the intensity of the testing to the character of the horse – none of this work should ever cause unnecessary distress to an animal), or it will dip a little and you'll see the flickering spasm of fasciculating muscles along the back.

Another test is right underneath the horse's tummy in the region of its sternum bone. It sounds brutal but you just dig your fingers in quite hard and quickly; a normal reflex response is for the horse to simultaneously drop its head and arch its back. If the horse is sore and tight it might not respond, or it may grunt and raise its back, but then hold it there and only let it back down back in painful small jolts.

Tail pull

Then comes the tail pull – and it's not the torture technique that its name suggests. First however I need to find out from the owner if the horse normally allows its tail to be raised – some just won't and will clamp down hard if you try, so for them the test is useless.

The reason for pulling the tail up and out is that it squashes the gluteal fascia and extends the sacral and coccygeal vertebrae. If there's a problem in those areas the horse will resist the tail pull. However, sometimes you may find the tail remains very flaccid, like a car's gearstick that has lost contact with the gears. This can indicate a serious neurological problem.

Despite its name, the tail pull is a very delicate procedure. The horse's natural reaction to its tail being pulled outwards in one direction is to pull against you in the opposite direction; go too fast and the horse can lose balance and fall. If the horse is really tight in one hindquarter it will actually enjoy it when you pull the tail the opposite way. However, because of the possibility of serious spinal cord problems, this test really does have to be done so gently, and never going beyond a critical point.

I'm now down to the last two parts of my assessment – muscle palpation and measuring any swelling.

Muscle palpation

Palpation can look like some kind of new-age hands-on healing but it is a diagnostic procedure that requires tremendous knowledge and skill. You're using your hands and fingers as eyes, feeling what is going on in all the different muscle groups. In essence, a healthy muscle at rest feels like a loaf of freshly cooked bread. It has a springy resistance when you palpate it between your fingers and run your hands up and down. A traumatised muscle feels more like a stale loaf with lumps of wood in it – a bit of sponginess and then you hit a hard layer. And in the case of muscle spasm, when you try to do a massage rolling technique where you pull the skin towards you and then roll it back, you find the skin and muscle are literally solid and inseparable.

A healthy horse will usually enjoy careful palpation and just stand there, but if there is any damage the horse may feel or anticipate discomfort and react accordingly.

Swellings

Finally I need to measure any swelling by comparing good and bad joints. And this will also help me to spot any muscle wasting. I can also examine what type of swelling it might be – soft swelling that feels like a soft jelly, effusion where pressure on one point makes the swelling pop out at another point, or blood effusion which feels a lot more springy and is hotter than tissue effusion (and gives the horse a lot more pain too). And if it is an older injury, I may notice that the soft jelly is beginning to set like concrete as it turns into scar tissue.

One final piece of work, when relevant, is to examine and assess any current wounds. Some injuries can't be effectively sutured – for example if the cut is over a joint and the movement keeps opening up the wound – and these may need to left to heal naturally by granulation. And that's where my laser comes in useful, speeding up the circulation to the area and minimizing scar tissue.

*

And that's it! My report then goes to the vet to help inform a treatment plan; and the owner, being present during the assessment, is much better informed if required to play a part in that treatment. And my report, like any other important document, remains safely filed for at least seven years as a record of a medical process.

On a final note, if you can see how thorough this is and why it provides such useful diagnostic information you'll also appreciate how frustrating it is that still, even now, proper equine physiotherapy can be undervalued or even unknown – to some horse physio is little more than massage and aromatherapy. And of course these are useful but there is so much more that chartered physios can do. Please help spread the word...

My description of the assessment process will, I hope, have made it really clear that there is any number of things that can go wrong with a healthy horse. And this means that physiotherapy is in no way the formulaic treatment that it may sometimes appear to be. Having said that, specific anatomical areas are prone to particular problems, and in this chapter I'd like to focus on a few of these and give you some insight to how physiotherapy fits into the overall care. And in some of the more detailed case descriptions in the chapter that follows I hope to convey how the whole process can be one of first discounting what the problem is not, before pinning down what it actually is – and even then can it require a mixture of scientific rigour and experienced gut instinct.

Foot problems

There is actually little that physiotherapy can do to help treat these cases. Far more important is a good farrier, and during my career I've been fortunate to watch some excellent farriers at work (I mention them in the Acknowledgments). Physios can offer the 'luxury' of using laser light to help heal an abscess, for example, but in my experience a good farrier will help to prevent this type of problem in the first place.

We're not entirely superfluous however and can offer some valuable diagnostic input. The vet can obviously use X-ray to examine hooves and pasterns in close detail. But sometimes they want to see a slightly bigger, more inclusive picture. The physio can help to flag up any imbalance in the hooves, their shape and the weight-bearing surfaces as well as limb conformation – sometimes observing and examining the horse in situ and on the move like this reveals more about the actual problem. And you will remember from the assessments that it's quite possible that the initial identified area is not in fact the source of the problem;

so the physio inspection helps to deliver a broader but connected perspective than a localized X-ray can give.

Fetlock problems

As with feet, the physio has only a limited toolkit for fetlock work, but it's a useful one nonetheless.

Ponies and horses with *windgalls*[11] can be helped using ultrasound, laser, electromagnetic therapy or cold water/ice/cryotherapy with pressure bandages. However, the success of these is somewhat dependent on the underlying cause, such as a conformation problem, awkward movement, concussion, or even obesity.

The same treatments can be used where a horse has effusions to the fetlock joint caused either by its kicking itself or brushing or hitting a fence. However, if there is an accompanying open wound, with a risk of infection or bleeding into the joint, it really needs full veterinary intervention.

In cases of *degenerative joint disease*, OCD (osteochondrosis dissecans[12]), *sesamoiditis*[13] or general wear and tear, physiotherapy can help to relieve the pain and inflammation but, again, full treatment also involves veterinary intervention and the all-important expert farrier.

Tendon and ligament problems

If any problem is suspected with tendons and ligaments, the first port of call must be the vet who can use ultrasound scans for very efficient diagnosis and to indicate a likely timescale for recovery.

---

[11] A swelling of the digital tendon sheath
[12] ossification of soft cartilage cells
[13] pain associated with the proximal sesamoid bones

Physiotherapy can then help the recovery using R.I.C.E[14]., laser, M.P.T. and S.T. manipulation if needed, and also by prescribing appropriate exercise therapy where useful.

Knee and forearm problems

Once again it is essential first to consult a vet for correct diagnosis; and any puncture wounds will need veterinary intervention to avoid infection.

Physiotherapy can be useful if swelling becomes thickened and the soft tissue needs mobilizing.

Stifle joint problems

These could arise from something as simple as a kick but can still be very problematic. The horse might present with a large haematoma that can be resolved quite quickly; but if the swelling persists then cold hosing, ice packs, laser and P.e.m.e[15] can help. If problems continue there might be patella or ligament damage in which case veterinary advice is needed.

Locking stifles[16] can be very distressing to the horse. The causes are various – from certain breeds types to injury or weakness. Veterinary advice is essential, but following diagnosis the physio can help by prescribing some controlled exercise to help strengthen the quads, hamstrings and core muscles.

Another time when physiotherapy input is useful is when a horse knuckles slightly in circle work. Obviously the horse's back should be carefully examined as the possible source of the problem, but if

---

[14] Rest, Ice, Compression, Elevation
[15] Pulsed Electromagnetic Energy Field Therapy
[16] commonly misdiagnosed as general lameness, but actually the result of one of the ligaments in the stifle joint remaining hooked over a ridge in the head of the femur bone

it's a need to strengthen the muscles of the back and hind legs then some good quality flat work and lunge work can be very beneficial, along with raised trotting poles, bounces and grid work.

Hock problems

These come in many forms so good initial diagnosis is essential before administering treatment. A horse, for example, that has slipped with its leg stretched out behind, overextending the hock, might present with effusions or haemarthrosis[17] and would need careful checking for these.

At soft tissue level, *thoroughpins* (a distension of the tarsal sheath) and *bog spavins* (inflammation from fluid swelling on the hock joint) can be treated with the usual range of cold-hosing, ice, pressure bandages, ultrasound, laser or P.e.m.e., providing they are mostly cosmetic. There may however be an underlying pathology relating to breed type or just to obesity. With bog spavins, it's sensible also to X-ray to see if there is any bone spavin, which can be treated by the vet or using P.e.m.e or short wave diathermy.

The same treatment options (cold hosing, etc) can work well for *curbs* (swelling in the plantar tarsal ligament) providing the swelling is soft. I've encountered many cases of curbs caused by the horse having had to pull itself out of very deep going, and suffering acute pain and swelling. However, it often indicates a conformational fault due to weak and upright hocks, in which case the problem may never completely disappear. Curbs can also cause the Achilles tendon to come off point of the hock; in these cases physio can only really help to manage the swelling, and again there may be an underlying mechanical fault that cannot be resolved permanently.

---

[17] bleeding into the joint spaces

Today's modern dressings mean that physio input may not be so necessary with wounds, but I still occasionally treat wounds to the hocks. Open wounds to the front of the hock can break down even if sutured; laser and other wound management can then help by speeding up the healing process. Puncture wounds to the hock can be especially nasty if there is any penetration of the joint capsule. Obviously veterinary intervention is required to manage any infection, but if the puncture area can be left open as a drainage outlet then laser is useful in speeding up circulation and getting the infection moving.

Shoulder problems

Shoulder problems can be very problematic and hard to diagnose. The most severe include avulsion[18] injuries to the brachial plexus, which causes paralysis (*Sweeney Shoulder*) to varying degrees sometimes with no recovery.

Fractures from trauma occur commonly from horses kicking each other in the field or running into gateposts. Muscular injuries can be caused by the horse rearing up and going over backwards (incurring neck injury as well). However, some shoulder problems arise as a result of injury or pain elsewhere. Some horses, for example, with a chronic front foot problem such as *laminitis* will hold themselves tense to keep the weight off the front feet. And soft-mouthed horses try to avoid contact with the bit by hollowing in the back and bringing the head back and in, leading to excessive strain on the shoulders.

Neck and back problems

This is perhaps the area where physios look the most for overlapping problems or difficulties arising from overcompensating for pain or stiffness. So I'd like to cover this in some detail.

---

[18] where a portion of cortical bone is ripped from the rest of the bone by the attached tendon

When you suspect an overlapping problem, you can't just go by the presenting symptoms; meticulous history taking, observation and examination are paramount to obtaining a full picture of what may be going on. And horses are just like people – if we have to work or sit in an awkward position and begin to ache on one side, we shift or compensate, developing similar problems on the other side. If you're a horse, you have four legs, not two, and often have a rider on your back, so the problems become multi-positional, generally compensating on the opposite diagonal. Hence on examination I might find that the opposite/diagonal part of the horse to the injured area is tighter and more painful – and you need to follow this algebraic puzzle carefully!

The terminology – near side, off side, fore and hind legs, left and right – can easily trip you up when you're trying to explain a problem or read a report, so I always use assessment diagrams to record clearly which part of the horse I'm referring to. If, for example, an owner has called me to a horse that is stiff to the right, I can show them accurately what is causing it: it may have more muscle on the offside of the poll and wither and can't bend round as easily; or it has a weak and stiff left hind leg and is tight at the left-side back of the saddle and hence resisting it; or perhaps its right hind leg is overdeveloped and the back is tight.

Neck problems usually arise from horses somersaulting in a rotational fall, or rearing up and going over backwards, and sometimes from a chronically poor way of going. And there's a very good manual therapy treatment that I've been really lucky to see and learn with David Gutteridge[19] over the past twenty years or so. David is a talented osteopath in both the human and equine worlds, and he uses a cervical spinal treatment that he gives to a sedated horse in the standing position – no mean feat, and in serious cases general anaesthesia may be required. I help to free up the horse to its limit or as much as possible, and David can then

---

[19] trained with Anthony Pusey and worked with vets Jane (nee Nixon) and Stuart Hastie

start to manipulate. With a following rest period of several days and then resumption of the correct exercises, this treatment can deliver fantastic results.

I remember David working with a show jumper that had fallen, had been fine for a month but then began hollowing and growing reluctant to jump. He was stiff on bending to the right and, after exercise, had a very wet sweaty patch on his near side splenius cervicis[20]. On examination he just couldn't turn his head to the left at all, and his back was sore on the right from compensating. So we treated the back, which helped a little, but he still couldn't turn his head. However, David could now proceed to manipulate the horse, with total full recovery.

Treating the back in acute cases can be really rewarding as it is generally some kind of muscle spasm and we have a whole battery of options to work with: massage, mobilization, soft tissue manipulation (many techniques for this, including the 'Ellis', the 'McTimoney', and the 'fascial release' techniques) as well as cupping, P.e.m.e., laser, ultrasound, light treatment, shock wave, electro-acupuncture, electrical stimulation... The list seems endless. And, with clear instructions for post-treatment care and our own follow-up care when necessary, the outcome is usually a happy horse and a happy owner – very satisfying all round.

Behavioural problems

This section has been a list of physical problem areas, but I also just want to mention behavioural problems as well (and you can also read more about where these sometimes take hold in chapter 17 which discusses buying and selling horses). Behavioural work forms a regular part of my remit and yet is an option that many owners are not aware of as they struggle with their uncooperative horse. Sometimes the horse is simply ill-natured or high-spirited;

---

[20] a muscle in the back of the neck

sometimes it is the owner who handles it badly; and sometimes the behaviour relates to the physical injury I've been treating where pain or discomfort has distracted the horse. Whatever the reason, assessing and diagnosing it correctly, along with a careful study of the animal's temperament, then provides an opportunity to work with it and improve it.

One of my earliest memories of behavioural work was when I was still at school – and as so often I have my father to thank for the learning experience. Looking back on memories of the two of us with horses is a bit like watching Laurel and Hardy, with me saying the famous line: "That's another fine mess you've got me into!" Dad's attitude to horses and their behaviour was somewhat simplistic and probably influenced by his wartime experiences when horses had to be efficient servants. He saw little value in trying to work with and around the problem to find a solution; they were simply horses and as such should be expected to function as required. And I can recall an illustration of this from when I was still at school, and which gave me a very useful lifelong lesson in being cautious and respectful (or maybe simply to use common sense) around feisty horses.

It concerned a pony belonging to a friend in the village. The pony was constantly misbehaving and bucking its owners off. Running out of ideas and patience, they came to Dad and me to see if we had anything to suggest. Dad immediately told me to get up on the pony, and so I dutifully obeyed only to be deposited onto the dusty ground. I was sent back up, and came back down in the same way. A few more times and I had had enough. "No, no, no!" I protested. "Put it on the lunge and give me a neck strap." And I was then able to mount and stay on while Dad sent the pony forwards. It was impossible, however, to tell if Dad was impressed by his first lesson in behavioural rehabilitation!

When talking about equine physiotherapy it might all seem to be about the horse and the physio – but we must consider the owner too! An effective and lasting equine physiotherapy outcome often requires teamwork, especially during any rehabilitation period after initial treatment.

Treatment and rehabilitation – who does what?

For simple problems, I may be able to do it all myself using a selection of hands-on techniques and specialist phsyiotherapy equipment. Often, however, a horse will require some post-treatment care to ensure the good work isn't undone. Where this requires continued expert skills (or where the owner is unable or unwilling to get involved) the horse will stay at the rehab yard as an inpatient. In other cases it is possible to send the horse home earlier to an owner who is ready to commit to weeks or even months of prescribed (and, if necessary, supervised) rehabilitation work with the horse.

However, getting involved as the owner can be tough, emotionally as well as physically. When a horse first shows signs of lameness, the instinct is immediately to rest the animal; and if the problem is muscular, this only makes things worse by exacerbating any weakness. Getting the physiotherapist in early (and the vet when necessary) means the horse can be properly diagnosed and prompt treatment administered to alleviate discomfort and begin the healing.

Treatment itself is not usually painful or uncomfortable; that would be unethical! You have an injured horse, already suffering, and any treatment must aim to reduce this as well as beginning a healing process. But once the treatment has done all it can, the rest comes down to rebuilding strength and resilience. There are no short cuts – the horse has to do some work if this is to happen.

And this is where it can be much easier for me at the rehab yard; I have no personal emotional investment in the horses I treat, just a professional and compassionate desire to do whatever I can to make them better. And because I've been doing this work day in, day out with thousands of horses, I can judge when pushing a horse further than it seems to want will deliver the improvement it needs. That can be a hard thing to ask of an owner with little or no experience of rehabilitation.

Some rehab can be as little as four or five days of careful lunging, something most owners would be capable of doing back at home. Sometimes, however, it can require a much more lengthy and involved commitment. Fortunately some of the owners I work with quickly grasp the techniques and become absolutely dedicated to their task – and their horse eventually recovers really well. But it can seem like a leap of faith at the beginning, especially if the horse has been allowed to rest before I step in.

I've recently been hugely impressed by one young lady, Jodie, whose dedication over three months helped her horse, Ted, regain optimum health and performance. Ted is a nine-year-old warm blood with no history of any injury that Jodie knew of. However, he clearly had a sore back; he is very long in his back, with an unlevel pelvis, and had become dramatically dropped in his back and buttock muscles on the off side. We examined Ted and assessed the extent of his weakness, and then gave Jodie some advice on lunging with a pessoa[21], schooling and general exercise. My former assistant Kate also gave Jodie some regular rehab lessons for the first eighteen months. Ted's back will always be prone to tightness due to his mechanical unevenness, but he is now out competing in jumping, showing, dressage, eventing and hunting! So it just goes to show what can be achieved, even in a

---

[21] A lunging aid like a pulley system that effectively creates a connection between the hind quarters and the bit to encourage the horse to be aware of and use its hocks

wonky patient, with ongoing exercise therapy (and owner dedication) to keep a horse strong where it needs it.

However, in case you're about to rush out and start lunging your stiff horse, stop. Exercise therapy is certainly the key to successful rehabilitation – but it must be properly prescribed, and even then it's no guaranteed magic bullet. There are several limiting factors: sometimes the animal just doesn't want to work with you or cooperate; sometimes, even with careful tuition, the owner doesn't carry out the therapy as prescribed, which can be ineffectual or even make things worse; and sometimes the damage is simply too great for the horse to return to its full time job.

As professional physios we also have the benefit of a rehabilitation yard, fully equipped for the tiniest adjustment in exercise therapies. So with inpatients we can offer the full spectrum of rehabilitative programmes. One end of the spectrum is for the horse that really does need to rest or take the weight off an injury; options include box rest and larger pens that allow walking but not galloping or larking about. At the other end of the spectrum are the options for hard active work – pole work and grid work, making use of different terrains (hard, soft, level, hilly undulating), and we can use water treadmills or even go walking in the sea. And for easy or moderately active work, there is walking in hand, using a horse walker, gentle riding, and using resistance such as weighted boots to increase leg strength. And within this broad selection we can also choose passive work that only impacts on certain joints such as the fetlocks, knees or hocks, and more active work for getting the fore and hind legs and neck moving.

Case studies

With hundreds of case stories to choose from I decided in the end to select just four that help to illustrate the assessment and treatment of some common injuries – 1) general soft tissue injury, 2) superficial tendon injury, 3) an overlapping shoulder/neck/back problem, and 4) a deep digital flexor tendon injury.

Please note, the figures used in these case notes relate to the particular machines that I used and may not reflect those found on other types of machines and instruments.

Case study #1: soft tissue injury

The horse

Age: 15 years
Occupation: hunter

History of presenting complaint (HPC)

- History of tripping a little in front when moving from one surface to another
- Feeling a little pottery in front
- One incident of losing footing down a hole and worsening symptoms since

Past medical history (PMH)

- Nil of note
- X-rays or scans[22] - nil
- Drugs – nil

On examination (OE)

Very big horse. Well put together but slightly loaded shoulder.

- From front: near fore hoof bigger than off fore
- From side: swelling between knee and fetlock medially and very slightly laterally up to back of knee, but reasonably clear

---

[22] NB this dates from more than 20 years ago when owners were reluctant to have their horses scanned. As well as being expensive (and this was Yorkshire after all...), X rays and scans were often over-exposed and the vets not always well trained to interpret them accurately.

lineation of tendons. Swelling measured as 1" and sited 1" below accessory carpal bone.

- On palpation: heat; effusion – soft in nature; tender to the touch/squeeze
- At walk: more or less sound
- At trot: lame; head nod

Conclusion

As no scans were available and not being able to diagnose a precise problem, it was judged to be a general soft tissue injury.

Treatment

- Rest
- Ice/cold
- Compression
- Laser therapy: daily on setting 'F' x 5 mins with the wide head on the medial and lateral aspects of the leg
- Electromagnetic therapy x 20 mins with the leg boot on the acute setting
- Instructions give to owner on how to apply ice/compression and how to use the machines. Warnings to reduce treatment to every other day if the leg becomes more swollen. Decision to review patient in 10 days

2nd visit

- Heat and swelling had reduced slightly (1/2")
- No untoward reactions to electrical treatment.
- Decision to review patient in 10 days

3rd visit

Horse still being bandaged and hosed.

- Swelling virtually disappeared, heat less
- Advised to use laser and electromagnetic for another 10 days, plus in hand walking for 10 minutes twice a day

4th visit

I discovered the owner had let the horse out to grass as the hunting season was now over – not ideal! But there was no recurrence of swelling or heat in the leg. I now worked out a rehabilitation plan that recommended:

- Stopping treatment and bandaging
- Asking farrier to examine foot balance to see if we could achieve more symmetry
- Not leaving the horse out all summer but instead embarking on regular walking, up to three miles and at least three times a week to keep the legs hard and keep mobilizing the scar tissue
- Some light schooling to keep the horse off his forehand as, at 15 years old, this wasn't helping his joints.

Outcome

I was still young, relatively inexperienced, and the owner was rather formidable; to be honest I didn't expect much of this rehabilitation to be done properly if at all. And there were no plans for further review. However, I learned that the horse returned to full work and hunting and continued for the next three seasons. My advice must have been followed!

Case study #2: superficial digital tendon tear

The horse

Age: 11 years
Occupation: Irish Draught hunter
Height: 17 hands

History of presenting complaint (HPC)

- Horse known to be lazy, and had inturned feet
- Horse was hunting and felt a bit pottery in front and reluctant to go forwards

- Possibility he had been cast[23] – had moved a hayrack and had a haematoma on his off hind in the groin area
- Swelling had been found in front near fore; vet scanned and found a superficial digital flexor tendon tear with a small hole (evidence of disrupted fibers)
- Vet's advice: box rest, foot care and rescan after 4 months. Drugs nil

On examination (OE)

- From front: boxy upright feet; pigeon toed
- From side: obvious 'bow' of tendon with medial and lateral swelling; heat; tenderness on palpation
- Swelling measured to be 2", cited 1" below accessory carpal bone

Treatment

- Rest, ice/cold hosing, compression
- Ultrasound 3MHZ, pulsed @ $0.5swcm^2$ for 4 mins each side and posteriorly
- Electromagnetic leg wrap x20 mins, on acute setting
- Decision to review in 10 days, and to recommend treating on alternate days if the leg filled

2nd visit

- Marginal improvement
- Swelling reduced to 1"
- Still sore on palpation
- Advise to continue treatment and review in 10 days

3rd visit

- More improvement
- No swelling of consequence and no heat or soreness

---

[23] Lain or rolled in stable and become stuck, unable to reposition or roll away

- Slight bowing
- Advised 10 more days ultrasound and EMT with increased U.S @ 3MHZ continuous @1.0wcm^2

  NB: *Physio readers may be horrified by this - but it works!*

4th visit

The client had turned their horses out as the season was over; treatment was stopped; symptoms had all but disappeared and the horse was sound.

I talked with the owner about balancing the feet and getting the horse off the forehand. He also wanted to use a blister to harden the horse's leg, an old fashioned method but I had no objection. We discussed a walking regime as a structured rehabilitation, and the horse returned to hunting the following season, making a relatively easy entry back to hard work.

Case study #3: overlapping shoulder/neck/back problem

The horse

Age: 5 years gelding

History of presenting complaint (HPC)

- Horse had reared and fallen over backwards on the lunge 12 weeks previously
- Received veterinary treatment; X-rays revealed close thoracic spines but they were not kissing; also overdeveloped in the brachiocephalics and with upside-down (or hollow) neck, having been worked incorrectly. And the possibility of mouth problems[24]
- Vet had treated by injecting steroids into the sacrioilac joints and thoracic spines

---

[24] These might typically be from teeth that had been neglected, or a large tongue and incorrect bits – or just a hard-handed rider!

<u>Treatment</u>

I prescribed one week of box rest followed by a rehabilitation programme at the yard:

Physiotherapy:

- Soft tissue manipulation/mobilisation to the neck, back and hamstrings
- Neck and carrot stretches
- Leg exercises/pulls

Exercise therapy:

- Weeks 1-2: in hand walking in tack x15 mins daily
- Weeks 3-4: *ditto* now x25 mins daily plus walking over poles and out on road
- Weeks 5-6: in hand walking x30 mins daily, ridden work walking x5 mins, pessoa alternate days at walk x5 mins each rein
- Weeks 7-8: daily work 30-40 mins; introducing trot on road/ in school on each rein; pessoa alternate days introducing trot each rein building up to 5 mins
- Weeks 9-10: daily work 30-40 mins; introducing canter on pessoa each rein building up to 3-4 mins, and on hacks and in school

I determined that after 12 weeks or on return to home, the rest of the programme would continue: more schooling work, pole work and grid work.

The horse improved well. He was a sensitive thoroughbred with a soft mouth so he would need a sympathetic rider, but he was discharged and managed well by a happy owner.

Case study #4: deep digital flexor tendon (DDFT) injury and to pedal bone on near fore

The horse

Age: 12
Occupation: 'Happy hacker'

History of presenting complaint (HPC)

The horse came to us as a veterinary referral with only a 20% prognosis of recovery. The vet prescribed a rehabilitation programme but with no lunging. Prior to coming to us the horse had presented with acute lameness; scans had revealed the DDFT injury. He was put on immediate box rest for three weeks, and corrective farriery was recommended to support the heels. Following the three weeks of rest, the horse came to us.

Treatment

- Began with daily horse walker x 10 mins on right rein (non loading leg)
- By week 4 this was built up to 30 mins daily plus 5mins under the saddle
- Weeks 8-9: now 20 mins under the saddle, mainly walking but with short bursts of trot (50-100 yards)
- Weeks 8-12: circle work added

Outcome

Despite the original gloomy prognosis, the rehabilitation was extremely effective. After 12 weeks the horse was discharged, sound and able to continue working with the owner.

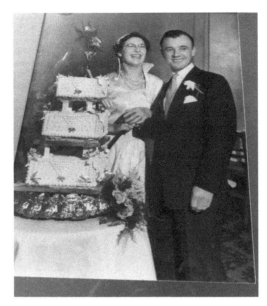

1. Mum and Dad on their wedding day.

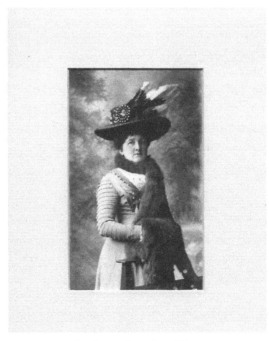

2. Great Grandma Riley.

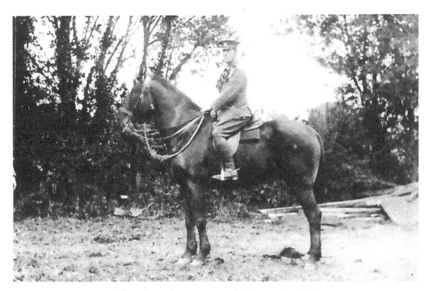

3/4. Grandpa Long on his horse,WW1.

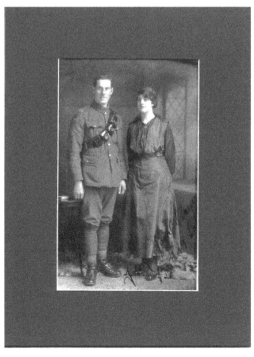

5. Grandpa Andrew Long and Grandma Louisa Long.

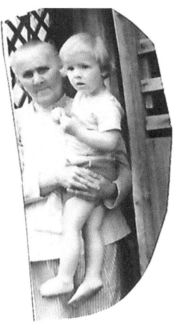

6. Grandma Skowronek with me.

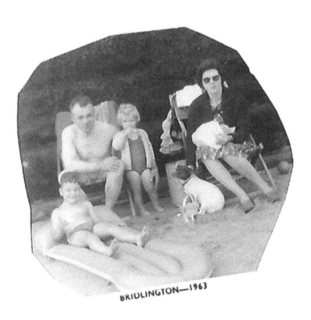

BRIDLINGTON—1963

7. Family time at Bridlington.

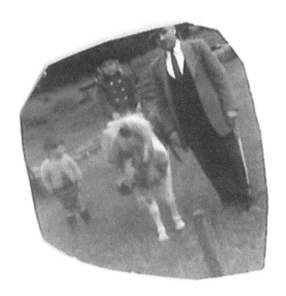

8. Toby my first pony.

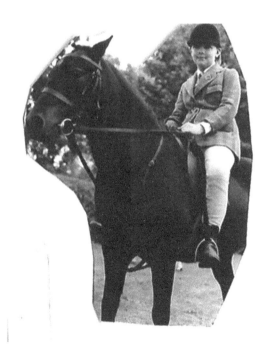

9. Gemini my second pony.

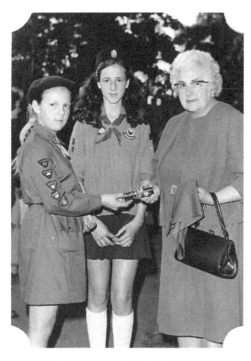

10. Katie the Brownie.(on left)

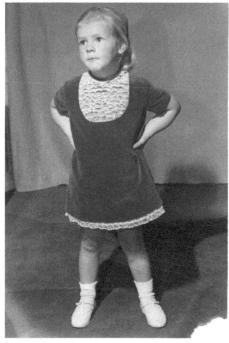

11. Little Miss. Precocoius!!!

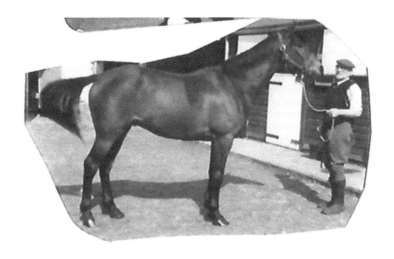

12. Randolph Greensmith and thoroughbred Whisthart.

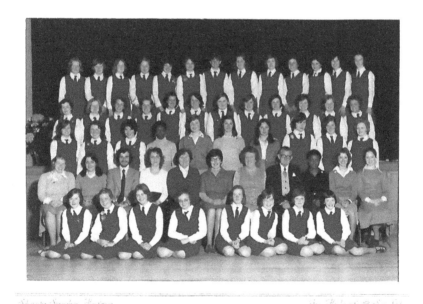

QUEEN MARGARET'S SCHOOL
ESCRICK — MAY 1976
Headmistress: Miss B. D. SNAPE, B.A., Hons. Lond.

13. School Photo me on back row 6 from right.

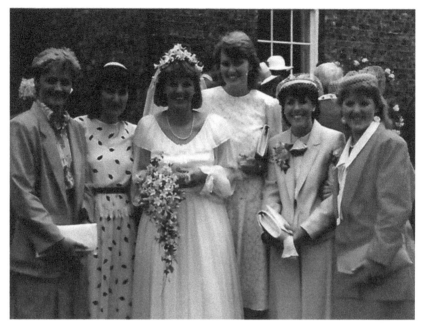

14. My wedding with my physio college friends.

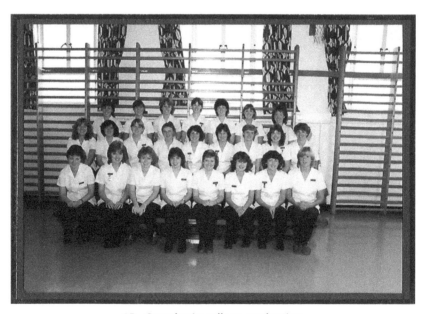

15. Our physio college graduation

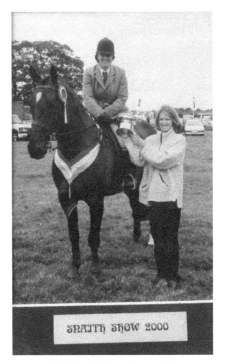

16. Lord Theodore and I.

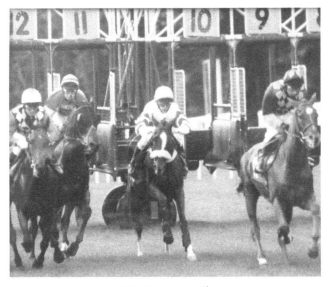

17. Portugese Lil.

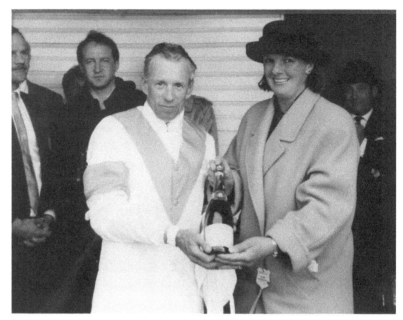

18. Presenting George Duffield with his prize as winning jockey of a race my husband had sponsored.

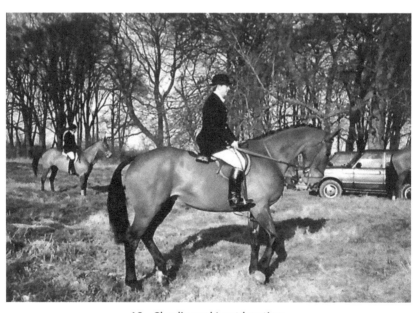

19. Charlie and I out hunting.

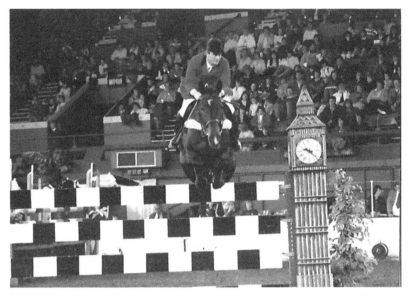

20. City Tycoon a horse we bred and sold that Robert Smith jumped at top level.

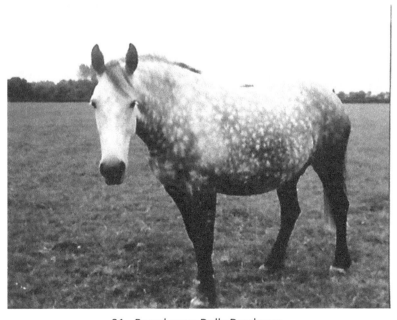

21. Brood mare Dolly Daydream.

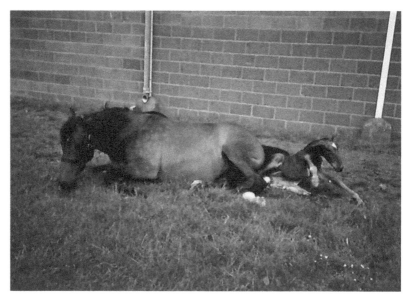

22. Brood mare Kasha having a foal.

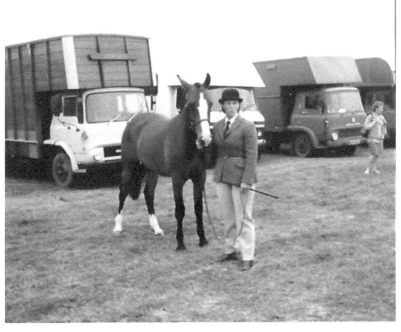

23. Bella the surviving twin who became the next broodmare.

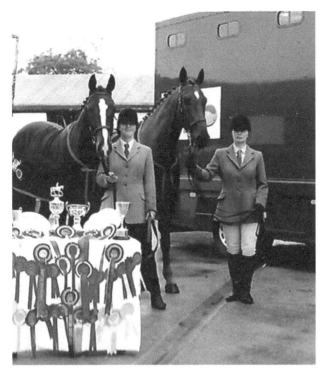

24. Classic Dancer and I, Lord Theodore and Jane Collins.

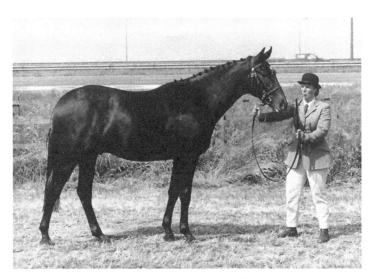

25. Patrick at 1 year old.

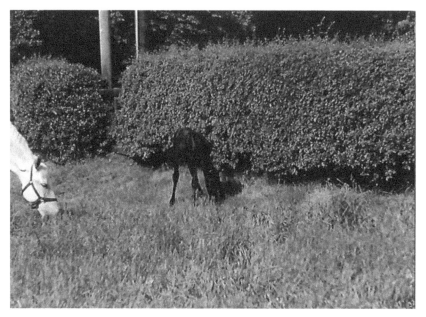

26. Patrick at 1 day with mum Penny.

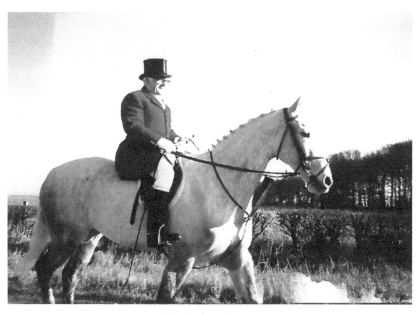

27. Dad on Penny.

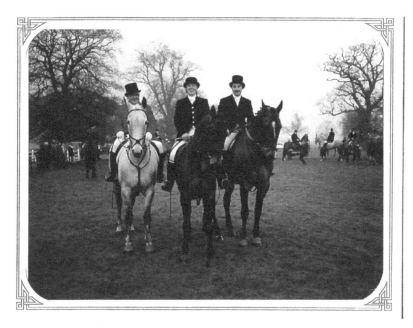

28. Dad, me and brother Richard on Penny, Sunny and Charlie respectively.

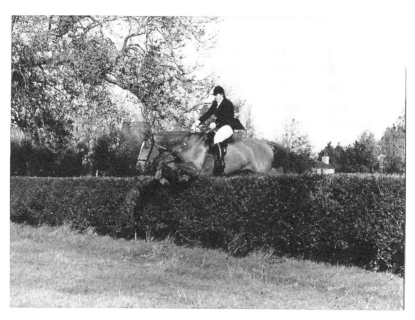

29. Rita and I hedgehopping.

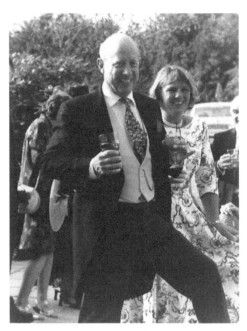

30. Godfrey and I at a family wedding.

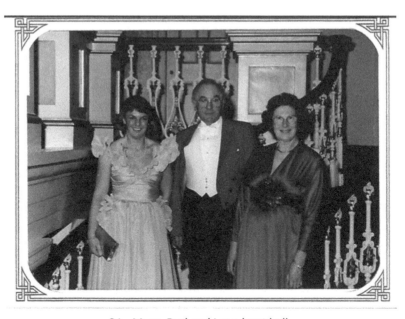

31. Mum, Dad and I at a hunt ball.

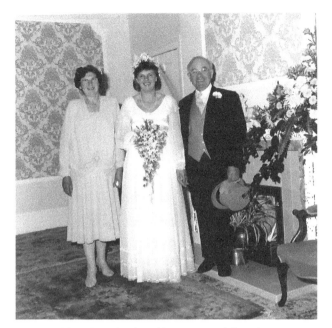

32. Mum, Dad and I on my wedding day.

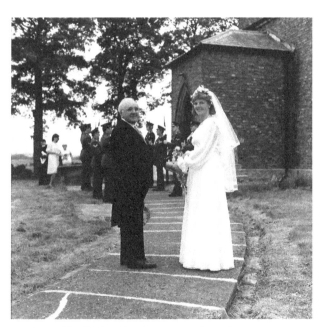

33. Dad and I about to go into church.

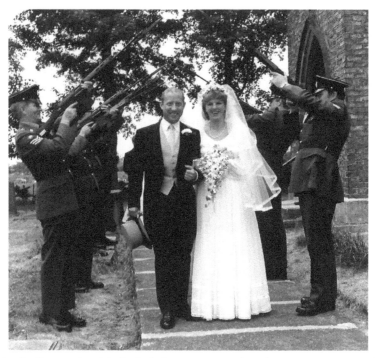

34. Godfrey and I with the lads from 219 squadron,(RLC, 150N Regiment).

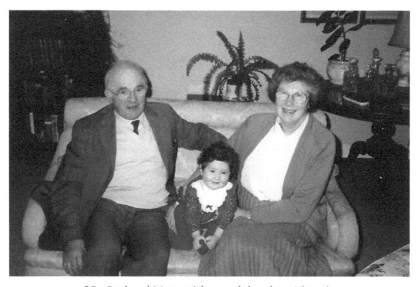

35. Dad and Mum with grand daughter Victoria.

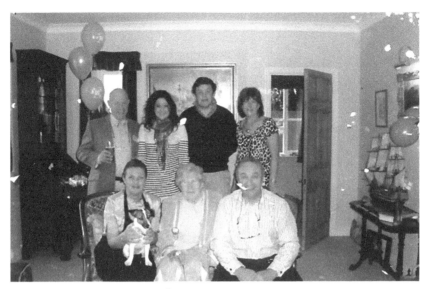

36. Mums 80th birthday party with the family.

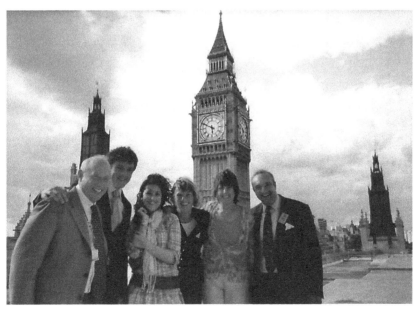

37. Godfrey and I with my family on McGees Peep.

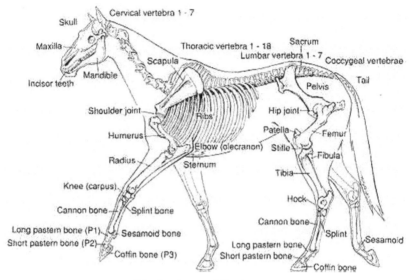

38. Anatomy of the horse.

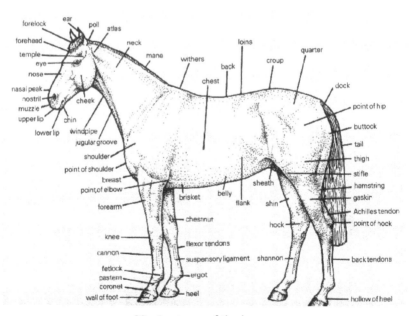

39. Anatomy of the horse.

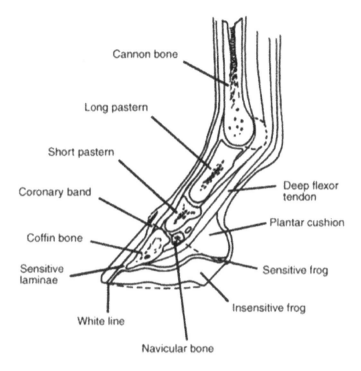

40. Anatomy of the lower leg of the horse.

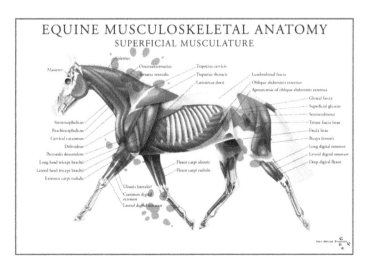

41. Superficial muscles of the horse.

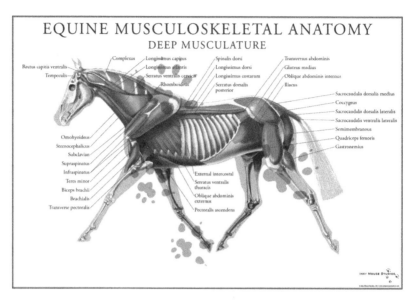

42. Deep muscles of the horse.

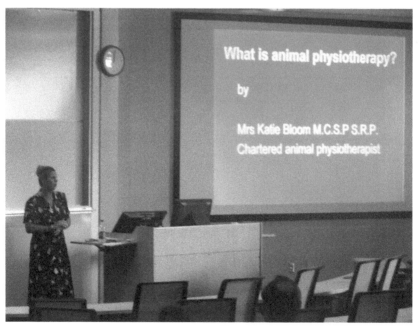

43. On a lecture tour in Alabama, USA at the veterinary College.

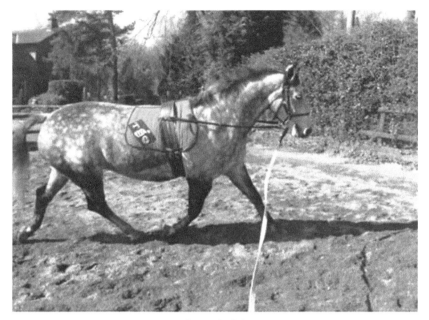

44. Before rehabilitation.

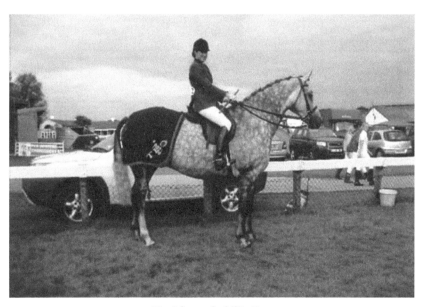

45. After rehabilitation.

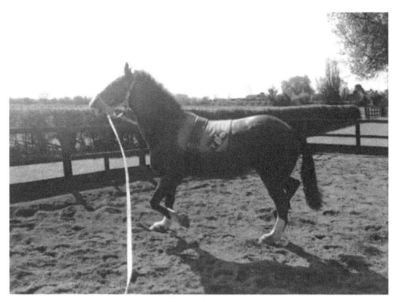

46. Before rehabilitation.

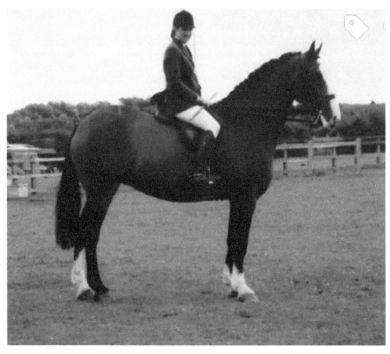

47. After rehabilitation.

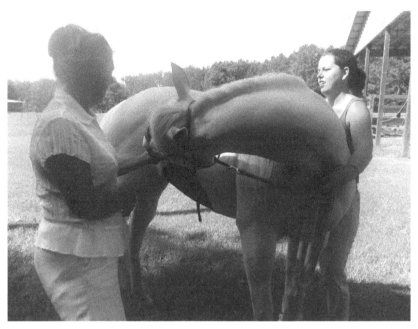

48. Assessing horses in Alabama.

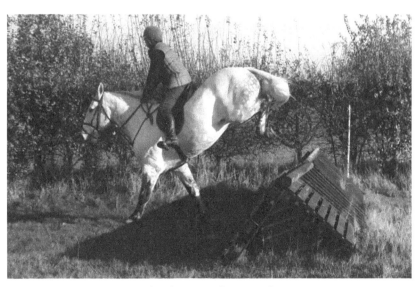

49. Schooling over fences at home.

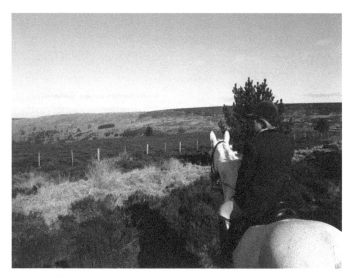

50. A lovely view from horseback in Yorkshire.

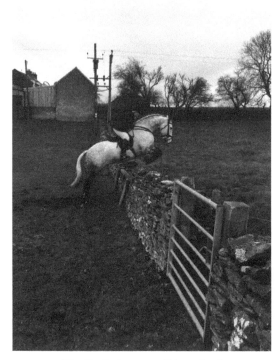

51. On Guiness, wall hopping!

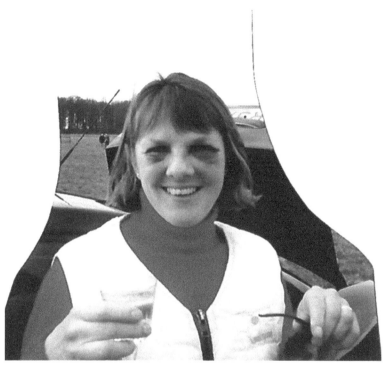

52. Black eyes from a glancing blow from a horse!

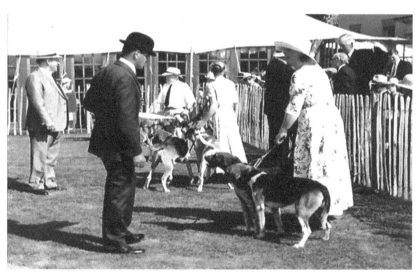

53. Hounds that I walked being judged by Wiliam Deakin.

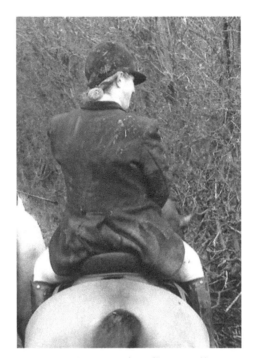

54. Oops a rather dirty coat!!

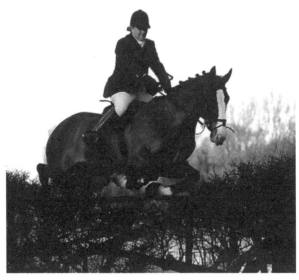

55. Hedge hopping on Ruby.

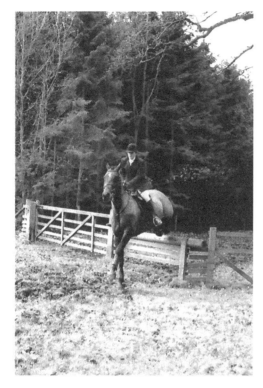

56. On Milo at Garrowby.

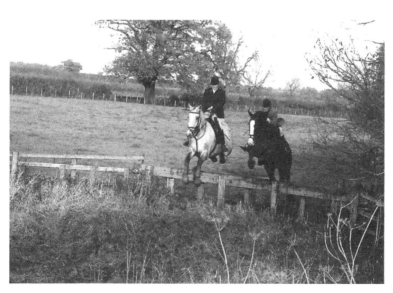

57. Delta and Ruby upsides at Leppinton.

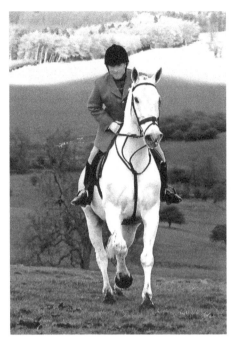

58. Mr. Cracker and Godfrey at Birdsall.

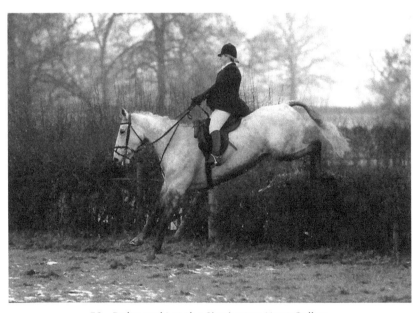

59. Delta and I at the Sinnington Hunt Gallop.

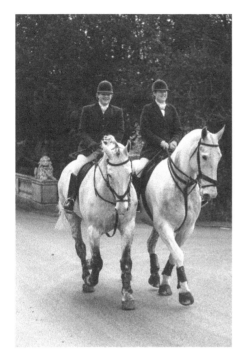

60. Guiness and Ted at Wynyard Hall.

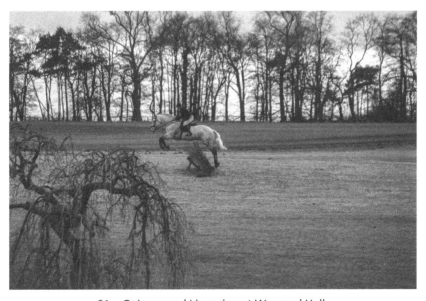

61 . Guiness and I jumping at Wynyard Hall.

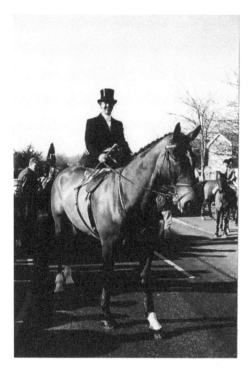

62. Maestro and I at the start of the Lucy Glitters Sporting Tour sideways.

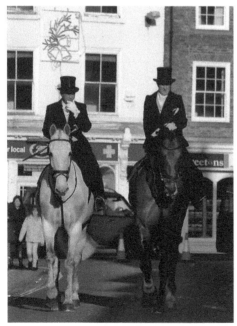

63. Looking elegant on New Years Day.

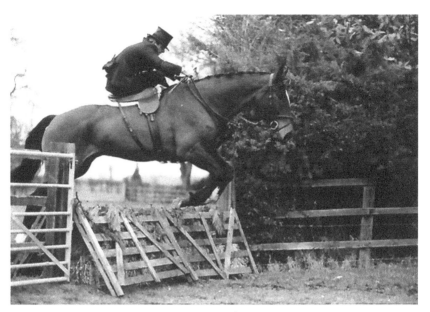

64. Jumping sideways.

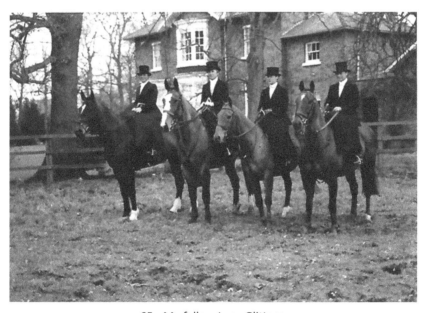

65. My fellow Lucy Glitters.

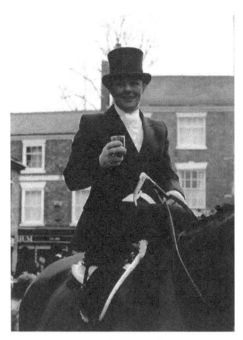

66. Sullivan and I.

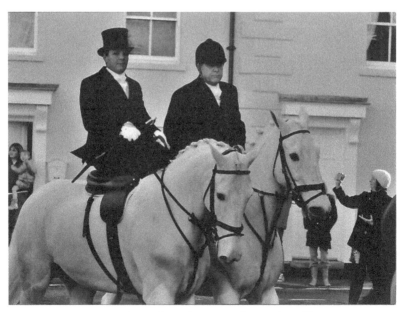

67. Murphy and I and Mr. Cracker and Godfrey.

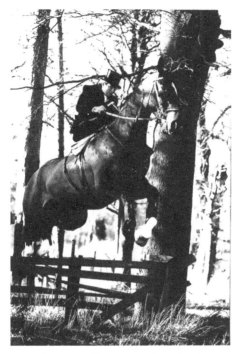

68. On the Lucy Glitters Tour jumping Maestro.

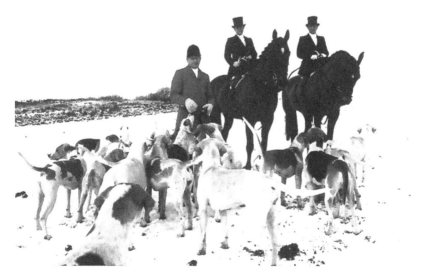

69. On Exmoor with the huntsman and Jane Collins.

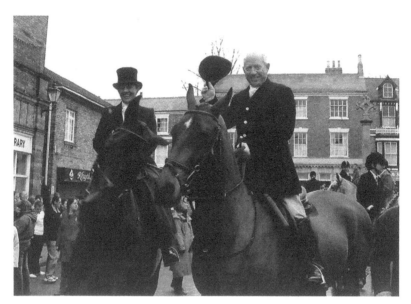

70. Godfrey and I with Milo and Sullivan.

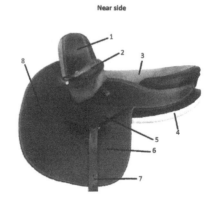

Near side

Fixed Head
Leaping Head
Seat
Wykeham Pad (made from pure wool Felt)
Safety Release Cover
Flap
Stirrup Leather
The Safe

71. Points of the side saddle, courtesy of Laura Dempsey an amazing saddler.

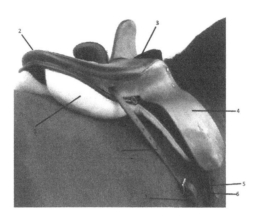

Offside

Serge Panel (flocked with pure wool)
Cantle
Cut-Back Head of the seat
Offside Flap
Overgirth
6   Girth
7   Balance Girth
8   Balance Strap

72. Points of the side saddle, courtesy of Laura Dempsey.

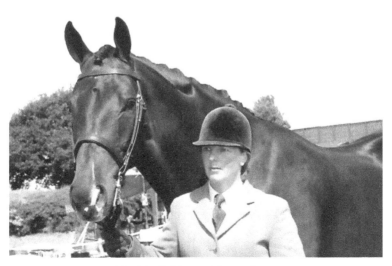

73. Mr Fielder and I at a show.

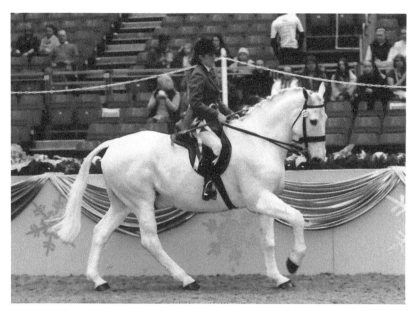

74. Mr. Cracker at Olympia in the Veteran Championships.

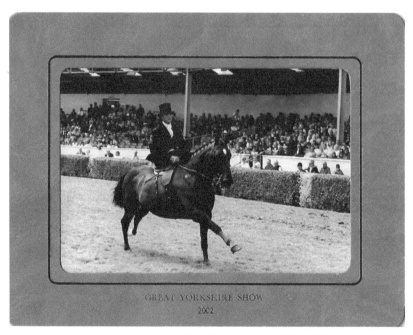

GREAT YORKSHIRE SHOW
2002

75. Lord Theodore and I at The Great Yorkshire Show.

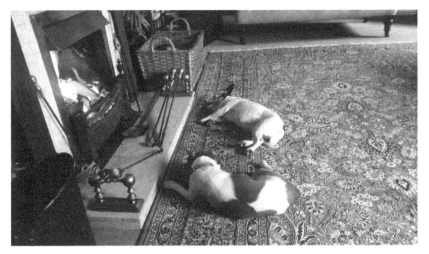

76. My Babies enjoying toasting in front of the fire.

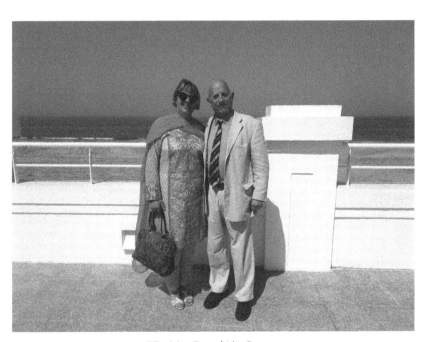

77. Mr. B and I in Oman.

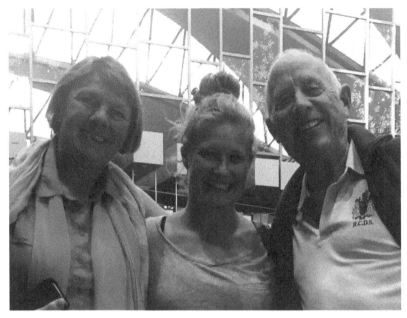

78. In Dubai with Ladies Jockey Joanna Mason, an amazing Yorkshire Lass.

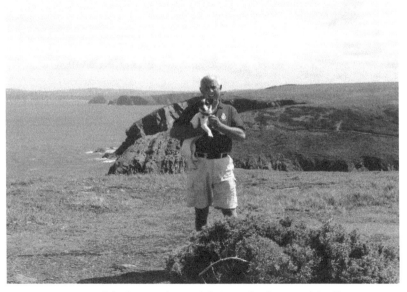

79. Holidaying on the Welsh Coast in the sun shine!!

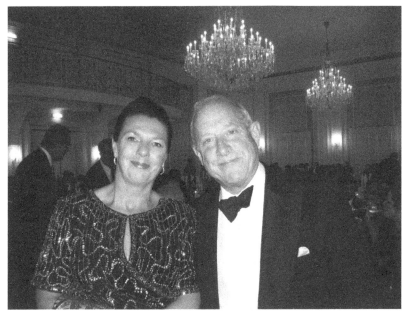

80. Ready to party!!

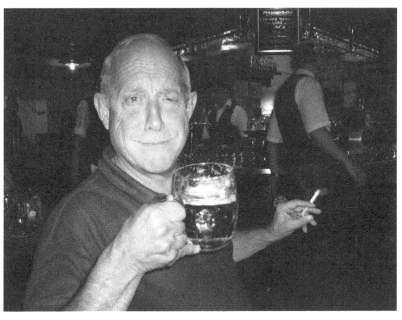

81. My husband having fun.

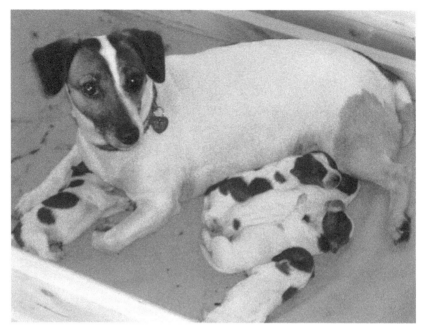

82. Chippy and her family.

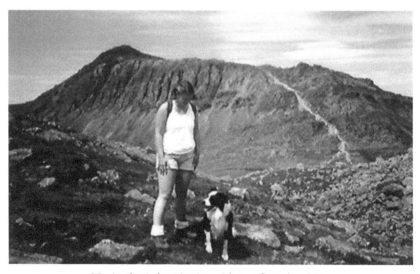

83. In the Lake District with our first dog Sam.

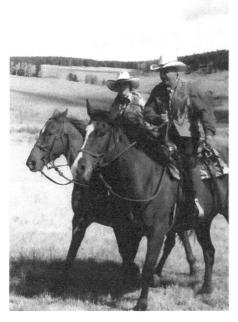

84. On a dude ranch in Wyoming(USA).

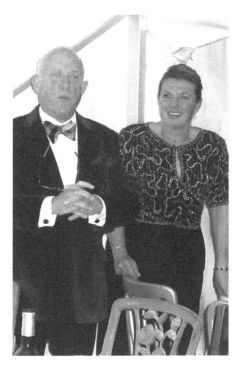

85. My 50th party.

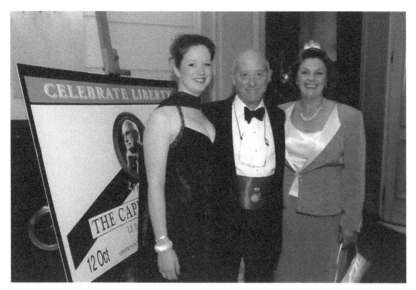

86. With Emma Lund, Godfrey's P. A.

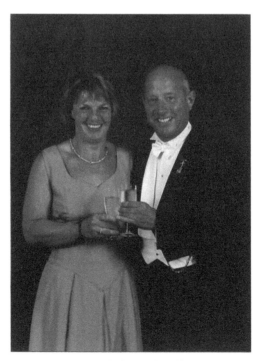

87. All dressed up!!

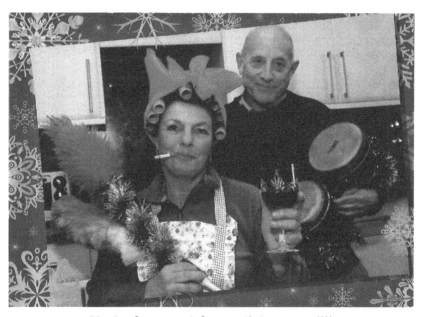

88. Our famous or infamous Christmas card!!!

SECTION THREE – TWO LEGS *PLUS* FOUR LEGS

CONTAINS:

Part Six – More fun with horses
(breeding, buying and selling, showing and racing)

Part Seven – Hedges, hunting, haute couture and husbands
(hunting; falls; sidesaddle touring; life with Godfrey)

In this part of the book we return to the more anecdotal reflections of my life, with a particular focus on the joys and the pains of equine activities. However, I must apologise to readers who prefer consistent chronology; of necessity I'll be jumping backwards and forwards in time, but will try to make things as clear as I can!

It was Kasha's first pregnancy. We all adored Kasha, the first offspring from Dad's beloved hunter, Katazynka. She was the sort of fantastic horse who does what it says on the packet – a superb jumper who competed at British Show Jumping Association (BSJA) events, and a dream to hunt.

We'd had no plans to breed from her, but circumstances took their own turns. Out hunting one day, Kasha had a nasty accident. She caught her hind leg down a land drain, cutting herself above the hock in the anterior tibialis[25], and almost slicing the leg off. Emotions were kept in check while we transported her carefully home, but once there I could no longer conceal my worry from my father. *"It's just a horse,"* he rebuked in his usual pragmatic way. *"She's not just a horse,"* I shot back, *"she's OUR horse!"*

A simple suture and primary intention healing were out of the question as the wound was too big and, situated just above the hock, would keep opening up under motion. Instead it would have to be allowed to scab over, then the scab picked off and the wound cleaned, left to scab again, and so on as it gradually reduced in size. Left to himself, Dad would probably have made the practical but sad decision that she must be destroyed. He was not a cruel man but his tough youth had nurtured an unsentimental attitude towards animals. However, he was up against my own potent mix of instincts - feminine, maternal, nurturing and stubborn – and I was also by this time a qualified physiotherapist. So, I knew there were other ways to treat Kasha; we hadn't run out of choices just yet.

---

[25] The muscle running down the 'shin' of the horse's leg

I called an acquaintance, Sarah Neville, who sold medical lasers and magnetic field therapy equipment. She helped rig me up and I began to treat the wound. We needed to encourage the wound to heal from the outer edges towards the middle – if you ever picked at scabs as a child, you'll be familiar with how it all works! So we decided to use laser therapy to increase the peripheral circulation, blood flow and speed up the healing process. Clearly a very healthy animal, Kasha responded really well while I repeatedly washed away the slough using a weak solution of hydrogen peroxide. But after healing she had a permanent limp – the injury had cut away a large amount of muscle – and so, unable to hunt or jump any longer, we decided to give her a new role as a brood mare.

Now, why the title to this chapter? By the time of this story we had already bred several horses; but did the saying, "Fools breed for wise men to buy" apply to us? Did we waste time and money trying to breed profitably, only for the buyer to dictate the terms? I don't think so, not least because we only sold our 'surplus' to those who knew what they were buying and had chosen the right animal for their needs. We kept our own horses to enjoy them, and we bred from them to enjoy their progeny; and as Kasha's story shows, if they were no longer fit for their original purpose but otherwise healthy, we didn't just get rid of them, not if breeding could give them a new focus in life. At one time, Dad had five brood mares and some forty foals, so it wasn't just a small hobby on the side but nor was it a foolish attempt to get rich quick.

So, what kind of person gets into horse breeding?

Well, not every horse owner wants to breed from their horse, but when you have ample fields and stables and a good supply of quality horses (still active or semi-retired) as we did, then breeding begins to make more sense. And once you start it can become an addiction governed by one of two possible drivers – money and satisfaction. And they don't often coincide. Our only interest was the satisfaction it brought. Our motivation was to experience creating our own lines of succession and to enjoy the results ourselves if we could. But as in any animal breeding, there were sad moments as well as joyful ones, and some tough decisions to be made. And as you just saw, Dad and I didn't always agree on how to make those decisions.

I think to most breeders it is a business first and foremost. It must make money, and to get the best profits you need to breed the best horses, pure and simple. Of course, this means that there will inevitably be foals that don't make the grade – one of the sadder aspects of the breeding world that I'll touch on shortly.

First let's just go back to the breeding at Wressle, and the two lines we produced from our initial foundation mares (see figures below):

Breeding Line 1

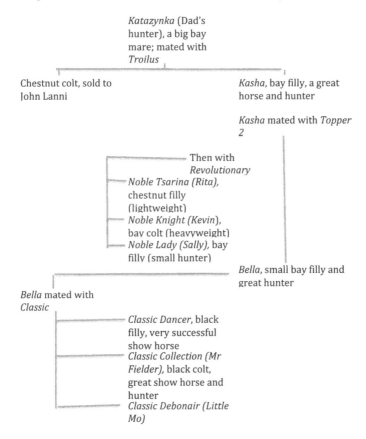

Breeding Line 2

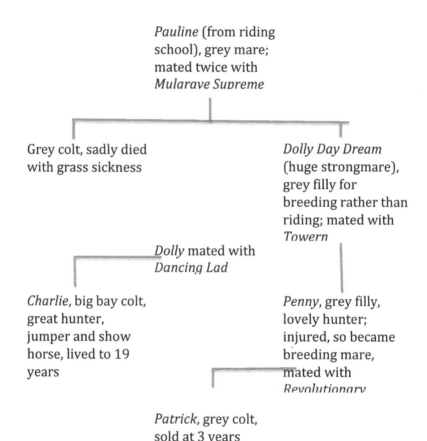

Pauline (from riding school), grey mare; mated twice with *Mularave Supreme*

Grey colt, sadly died with grass sickness

Dolly Day Dream (huge strongmare), grey filly for breeding rather than riding; mated with *Towern*

Dolly mated with *Dancing Lad*

Charlie, big bay colt, great hunter, jumper and show horse, lived to 19 years

Penny, grey filly, lovely hunter; injured, so became breeding mare, mated with *Revolutionary*

Patrick, grey colt, sold at 3 years

You can see here how all our breeding originated from two mares, Kasha's mother Katazynka, a big, strong, brave and intelligent bay and a really good hunter, and Pauline, a large horse from Dad's riding school. And with each new foal we were looking out for additions to our own hunting team or future brood mares as well as assessing for possible show potential.

Of course there were many youngsters that Dad sold. Some became successful in racing, point to point, eventing and jumping, including City Slicker and City Tycoon which competed internationally, ridden by Robert Smith, son of Harvey Smith.

And others were destined for more humble careers but Dad still assessed the potential buyers very carefully before agreeing to sell.

Finding the right stallions for the mares was, of course, crucial to a good outcome and a huge part of the challenge and enjoyment of breeding good horses. We were lucky that Max Abraham (and later his son David) kept many fantastic stallions not far away in Wilberfoss. One of his wards had been Mulgrave Supreme, a Cleveland Bay stallion belonging to the Queen. Given my Dad's immense patriotism, I'm not surprised he chose to pair one of HRH's finest with Pauline to start that line, but for Katazynka's the better match was deemed to be a brown colt called Troilus. And eleven months later along came Kashsa (Polish for Katie) who would become our first foundation mare.

Kasha popped out in early March, and for competition horses, the earlier the month the better. Age-governed classes go by the year of birth rather than the actual date, so for example a horse born in March 2012 is going to be that little bit stronger and more experienced than a 2012 class competitor born in July of the same year. Of course it was cold and snowy in the North of England, but we still managed to get mother and foal onto grass pretty soon. However, Kasha was also the type of foal every breeder dreads - a chestnut filly, about as stigmatized as ginger-haired women! But rather than use this as an excuse to sell her, as other breeders might have, I kept her. And I'm so glad I did. For a chestnut she was surprisingly trainable (many behave like divas) and matured into a really good horse and a good hunter.

Now, there are actually two tricks to successful breeding. One, as I've mentioned, is to find the right stallion; the other is to ensure a successful impregnation – and back then pulling off both tricks was still a bit hit and miss[26]. For one thing we didn't have the

---

[26] Acknowledgement must go to Jon Pycock's pioneering work in equine reproduction services that has done so much to reduce these uncertainties that we struggled with back then.

benefits of today's accuracy in charting the mare's fertility cycle. There were other unknowns to live with too, as we also lacked the new ultra-sound equipment that can detect twins early on. Horses don't carry twins well, and generally it's kindest to remove one twin when detected to give the other the best chance of survival. But without this modern tecnhology, we had no way of knowing there were twins until the birth or until the mare unexpectedly slipped them prematurely, by which time the damage had often been done.

This is exactly what happened when Kasha was mated with Topper 2, delivering twins eleven months later. One was a stillborn colt, more or less mummified in the womb, and the survivor was a tiny filly. The filly was very weak and struggled to suckle in the first hours of life. And so the stage was set for another duel between Dad and me. His down-to-earth view was that she would either live or die, and that was that. And totally the wrong thing to say to a stubborn Katie! Determined to do more than just watch and wait, I stepped in and milked Kasha so that I could feed the foal myself. The tiny little thing still couldn't stand but she latched on to the bottle and by bedtime, after a long day of doing this, she finally managed to suckle from Kasha. Dad, of course, was as thrilled as I was and we named the foal Bella. After that experience we were certainly going to keep her, and in her turn she became the next breeding mare.

Bella was a super horse. An endearing bay with an unusually broad pale white face, she was not beautiful – a bit of a runt really. And she wasn't the fastest either. But she was a reliable, kind and steady horse who gave everyone confidence, and a safe conveyance and jumper in the countryside. I spent many happy hours hunting on Bella, but gradually work demands began to limit my time for this and so eventually I decided instead to put her in foal.

This time the search for a suitable stallion took us to Josie and Steve Knowles at the Beechwood Grange stud. As often happens, the stallion provisionally earmarked for Bella, in this case one called State Diplomacy, didn't strike us in the flesh as the ideal match. So instead we went with a dark brown boy called Classic. As the story goes on to show, our hunch must have been a good one. It also illustrates why breeding and showing so often go hand in hand.

When you breed, and the result is a fine horse, it's not surprising that you want to show off the progeny via the world of horse showing. And there's a commercial benefit to this too, both for the owner when selling the horse and for the stud and stallion that helped produce such impressive offspring. Bella's first foal, Classic Dancer, was a lovely almost black filly with a white blaze. And Dancer really did dance! I showed her first as a yearling and she was soon winning hunter yearling classes far and wide. One of Dancer's proudest moments was beating nationwide competition at the national hunter show yearling filly class at Malvern. And of course, all of this reflected well on Classic and his stud reputation.

Dancer could have kept the breeding line going into subsequent generations, but my time was very limited and the rest of the family were no longer interested in breeding. Reluctantly I sold her, a decision I regretted, especially when I found out later that she had been bred from but had then been destroyed after an accident in the field. Such are the highs and lows of keeping strong breeding lines going.

Bella's next two, Classic Collection and Classic Debonair, I kept, and they did so well on the showing circuit that requests for Classic's siring now went sky high. If only I'd bought shares! Classic Debonair, aka Little Mo, was sold as a five year old, but Classic Collection – Mr Fielder, a black colt – went on to become a wonderful hunter and show horse, one of the best horses I bred.

You'll have seen there is another breeding line in the family tree, starting with Pauline, an unglamorous name for the riding school horse who, despite not being much use as a school horse, did possess the twin attributes of size and strength. And sure enough, paired with Mulgrave Supreme her first foal, Dolly, was also a great lump of a thing. But we saw something of real potential in Dolly, the makings a great hunter. And as we were still very much involved in breeding, we decided not to break her in but instead use her as a foundation mare to produce a good line of solid hunter horses with a lot of bone. Further down the line came Penny, another super mare who then suffered a hunting injury; she was not sold or destroyed but instead enjoyed a new lease of life as a brood mare. I think this once again shows that our primary interest was in our own experience of keeping and breeding horses rather than just making money out of them. Above all, our whole approach was to let each horse develop and show its strengths and then for us to try to facilitate those accordingly.

So, what of the wider world of breeding beyond the gates of the Wressle yard? Well, I certainly don't want to upset anyone or invite a law suit, but there are some very sad practices in this world, and I just want to reflect on one – the 'failures' that no one wants.

I've said already that breeding and showing go hand in hand. And I really admire those who do it – you need a lot of horses and will see many generations come and go, while never forgetting your first horse. And you must expect to wait a good four or five years before your new horse can show off its paces and ability in the ring. That's a big investment and a long delay before, with luck, the prize money starts to roll in. But of course, the real financial gain is in the stud provenance of your trophy-winning horse.

So what happens to the newly-bred horses that don't make the grade? Well, most are weeded out early on with clearly identifiable problems – those with turned out hooves for example. Rejected by the stud and professional breeders, these are now completely at the mercy of the dealers. A few horses, the lucky ones, will land on their feet and find owners for whom they are perfectly suited; others just continue being tried out, found wanting and sold on. And with each successive 'failure' their value goes down. Life can be pretty rough for lower-quality horses; it's not good. And as the next chapter reveals, there is more to say about this and the pitfalls of unscrupulous sellers and naïve buyers...

"Warrant it? I wouldn't even warrant it's a horse!" (Surtees)

I've never been involved much in buying and selling. But I've come across all kinds of sellers – and all kinds of buyers too. The perfect match between horse and human comes when both seller and buyer work together to find the right animal. But this isn't easy when the buyer is inexperienced and the seller less than scrupulous.

Nonetheless, with all our interest in breeding, riding, hunting and showing, why didn't we ever get into selling?

The horses we did sell from Wressle were mostly young and neither broken, ridden or trained (i.e. not yet 'produced' in equine terminology). So in a way they were blank canvases; we couldn't and wouldn't promise anything to the buyer beyond the provenance of the horse and the possible characteristics that may bring. And of course horses sold like this cannot command high prices, so it was never a money-spinner.

When you sell a horse you give up any rights to it and to its wellbeing. And that can be tough. Many horses that are sold end up being very happy with their owners, but even with the best-intended owner things can go wrong – and I've never wanted to be responsible for selling a horse into an unhappy life. For a successful placing there must be a partnership between human and animal, one that can grow into mutual trust and affection. It's not unlike a friendship between people. But we don't often give the horse the chance to decide who it likes and who it doesn't – until it's too late.

Both parties in the partnership are capable of an instinct, a feeling about each other on first meeting. But of course it is not an equal relationship; the horse does not possess the human's capacity for insight and for adapting its own behaviour. Some horses, for example, can be peevish by nature and need a firm hand to command respect. Equally, some people are peevish, but can a horse fully understand this? Of course not. So in my view when things go wrong early on, the onus can be firstly on the owner to adapt and only then on helping the horse to adapt.

Sadly this often doesn't happen. People have unrealistic expectations of how their new horse should behave and so they rarely blame themselves when things go wrong. They can also underestimate the lasting impact those earliest interactions between new owner and a young horse can have on the relationship. And the first casualty from this can be trust. Without trust early on, no animal will eagerly give its attention to its owner or trainer. Why should it when it feels unconfident of what might happen? And without trust, everything soon begins to unravel.

Problems in horses, as in people, tend to multiply if left unaddressed. So a young horse with a bad experience with its first owner may carry that on to the next owner and the next. It's not impossible to work with a legacy of poor handling and improve the horse's behaviour, but you need to fully understand the depth of distrust it will have acquired along the way. In fact, this is the real tragedy for many poor horses because the best window of opportunity is when they are still young, just newly broken and not very used to being ridden. The greatest care and empathy is needed to settle this young horse in.

So, an unsound horse needs special skill that new owners often lack; but also a sound horse, suddenly rehomed to an inexperienced owner, can just as quickly lose confidence. The outcome is always some degree of the same – an unpredictable animal; and all because, when selling a horse, you have little chance to assess and judge the potential new owner. Even the best sellers have to rely to some degree on trust; and once the transaction's done there's no going back. So, that's why I've never taken much to buying and selling horses. *Caveat emptor*[27] always seems a bit too one-sided to me – where's the warning to the seller about the buyer?

In addition to the horses I've bred I have acquired others over the years, but they mostly came to us first as patients or in need of reschooling and trust-building. I've always been very lucky to have skilled and talented people around me and so we usually manage to turn most of these horses round and then train up the owner to continue the good work; but sometimes the owner is so exhausted and their morale so low by the time they come to us that, after a short break from the horse, they admit they don't really want it back, improved or otherwise.

We've also occasionally worked with horses that we've come to judge as too risky or unfixable to go back to their owner. Some can make real progress with us, outstanding progress in fact, but the moment you drop your guard the old behaviours bounce back. These horses need to be constantly in a disciplined environment, and so they have often ended up with me for the rest of their lives.

So, that's my own experience, and you can see that I'm very wary of how easily things go wrong. But I can offer a little more to help to any enthusiast thinking of buying a horse. Let's consider the three principal parties – the buyer, the seller and the horse itself.

You can get some fundamentally bad animals just as you can with people, but let's assume the horse, incapable of guile, is the innocent party. And let's also assume that with the buyer the only common flaw is naivety. That just leaves the seller…

Sellers come in three main guises – the breeder, the producer and the dealer (and a fourth option would be via the horse sales). So what are the essential qualities in good examples of these?

Well, the good breeder is selling an unbroken horse but with some information about the breed line; so it's down to that blank canvas

---

[27] Let the buyer beware

again, but if you go on to ensure the horse is produced properly you may be fortunate and find you have a very sound animal. The good producer who is selling will have worked the horse slowly and methodically, and you should expect a settled head and a sound horse. The good dealer will take time to understand your equine experience and what you're looking for, and should have a good selection and be able to help you choose. And the fourth option, the horse sales? Unfortunately there isn't really such a thing as a good or a bad sale; the horses on offer will be largely unknown and may or may not be warranted, so really you are just gambling in the end.

Now, there are a great many good horse sellers. I've been fortunate to know some over the years; I've hunted with them, treated their horses, enjoyed their company and watched as they sell some truly magnificent horses. But how do you spot – and avoid - the dishonest or unreliable ones?

You need your wits about you – and to be frank it's not that different from buying a second hand car. It's not uncommon for sellers to assure you that the horse you have your eye on is the best horse you could possibly find. They'll say it will do everything you want, from galloping to jumping to doing the crossword and baking a cake. Some, however, will give you a tiny chance to dig deeper; they'll say things to you in a particular way to give the more experienced buyer the chance to ask more pertinent questions. Or they'll word it all so that their testimony remains open to interpretation. Either way they're off the hook if you try to go back to complain. And even if you know what to ask, it can still be incredibly difficult to get the information you want when buying. Some dealers will (deliberately or otherwise) bombard you with information until your head feels it will explode. Others can be rather standoffish and rude and leave you untended.

There are worse practices. Some sellers have been known to give the candidate horse a small sedative. You try out the horse and of course it behaves calmly with no histrionics of any kind. So you buy him, get him home, the sedative wears off - and your Dr Jeckyll turns into Mr Hyde. But of course you have no comeback; nothing can be proven, as the sedative will be long out of the horse's system unless blood samples were taken at the time or purchase.

I'd like to think, however, that on the whole sellers get an unfairly rough hand in certain parts of the equine world. Most are good people with a job to do and a living to make; and they try to do that as responsibly as they can. You will know you have found a trustworthy seller if he/she takes the time to find out about you. They will know that a good purchase decision is one that will promote trust between horse and owner and will forge a happy relationship.

A final cautionary word to buyers: even the seller with the greatest integrity can be fooled or overwhelmed by a buyer's insistence on a particular horse. And as a buyer it is almost inevitable that your thinking will be coloured by your emotions. You see two horses, one stunningly handsome, the other rather plain. And the responsible and knowledgeable seller has talked with you and understands your experience and your ambitions for your horse - and had deduced that the plain one is the only option. You, however, are hopelessly in love with the handsome one, and nothing will budge you. If you go home with that horse and things go wrong, you have only yourself to blame. So whose fault is it? Well, the seller has bills to pay and a family to keep, and it's clear you're not going to abuse the animal; so if you were that seller, would you refuse to sell the handsome horse? Probably not. But remember that a good seller will try very hard to match rider to horse – and they have a lot more experience than you will. So listen carefully and let your head guide your choice, not your heart.

If you were to ask me what was my most enjoyable equine pursuit, the answer without any hesitation would be hunting. So it may seem strange that it was showing, and not hunting, that became so obsessive as almost to threaten the marital bliss of the Bloom household. Showing horses is something that can entrap any breeder or rider, but without our horse shows we would lose a huge focus for almost every aspect of the horse enthusiast's world. I suppose the challenge is to keep control over it before it takes control of you.

More on this in a moment, but let me first clarify that I think horse showing is a healthy and necessary interest for keen horse people. It gives owners a goal, months ahead, for getting the horse into the best condition. It helps to maintain standards of breeding and training. And surely, you might ask, it's a way of bringing people together in a convivial manner to support and nurture their common interest? You'd think so wouldn't you - but if the compulsive and competitive bug catches you, watch out!

Showing was my idea to begin with, not Dad's. In fact he was dead against it at first, just couldn't see the point of it. He knew his horses and what they could do; he didn't need public endorsement or fancy rosettes and cups to validate them. But we had bred the wonderful Charlie just a few years earlier, and I persuaded Dad that we should give it a go. What clinched it, I think, was Godfrey. I was working in Hull at the time and still living at home, but with my future husband already on the scene I think Dad could foresee the time when I wouldn't be around so much. And he saw the potential for our showing adventures to provide him with exclusive father-daughter time.

Charlie was a really big lad, three years old, and had till now thoroughly enjoyed just doing his own thing in the field. So first I had to get him used to a different experience – being handled and tied up, having tack put on, being moved over this way and that, being lunged, being brushed – generally learning good manners for when he was out and about. And this is one of the great benefits of showing; it provides both the motivation and the structure for educating a young horse. But boy is it hard work too!

We had some good successes showing Charlie, both in hand and ridden, but he was also a good jumper and hunter trialler. He eventually retired from the show circuit and became my brother's hunter. He was also one of my early equine physio successes. Aged sixteen he sustained a check ligament injury. He first had box rest before undergoing ultrasound and magnetic field therapy. Slowly but surely we rehabilitated him with a lot of road walking and trotting, and he remained sound for the rest of his life, hunting until heart failure got him aged nineteen.

I did all the hard work preparing and grooming the horses for shows, and Dad shared the driving and made himself useful holding the horse between classes. Fair enough, it was all my idea after all. But gradually people began to come up to him to admire our horse and ask if it was his. And when the horse was sporting a red rosette, I could tell Dad was proud even if he did his best to conceal it. I could also tell that he was as frustrated as me when we didn't do so well. Submitting your horse, or indeed any animal, into a competitive show is like putting your baby on display, to be assessed and judged. I still show my Jack Russell occasionally, and if she isn't given first place I'm really gutted.

So, off we'd go, the two of us in the Land Rover with one or two horses in the trailer, doing the Yorkshire circuit (shows such as Tockwith, Driffield and Syke House) and sometimes venturing beyond. And you get to recognize the same old faces at different shows; but you don't necessarily get to talk to anyone, not properly. It's very competitive and a bit bitchy, dominated by women. You learn to recognize the judges too. Most of our showing was at events organized by the Hunter Improvement Society (now renamed Sport Horse Breeding of Great Britain). It's all run very well and since the judges are, in a way, ambassadors for the society they need to be respected and knowledgeable. They used to be drawn from the great and the good of the hunter world but more recently the job has been opened up to people from within the show world's competitor community as well.

I think the most fun I had showing in hand was with Bella's colt foal by Classic – show name Classic Collection, and stable name Mr Fielder (after a corpulent local builder, Dave, who always referred to himself as Fatboy Fielder. Tactfully we didn't reveal to Dave the true reason for the name, saying instead that it was "because the horse was such a handsome dude!"). In his yearling days of showing, Fielder could be a bit cheeky; but with experience came maturity – he grew to love it and learned to show off just through the way he stood and moved, as if to say: *"Hey, look here, look at me!"* He was also successful in his ridden show career, disproving the common belief that a good in-hand horse will never succeed in ridden classes. In fact, he did more than disprove them; he went on to qualify for and achieve minor placing in lightweight hunter and ladies' sidesaddle classes (in the good old days when silk top hats were still allowed) at the Royal International Horse Show and the Horse of the Year Show. Finally he followed Charlie by 'retiring' to a long life of great hunting.

I had great fun doing some judging myself at a lot of unaffiliated shows, and I decided to take it further by putting myself forwards as an affiliated judge (although in the end time constraints prevented me from becoming a panel judge). For this, you had to follow a well-worked out process, beginning as an apprentice, then graduating to probationary judge before finally becoming a qualified judge. This rigour is really important, not least because show results can have a major impact on a horse's value; make the wrong judgement on the day and a shadow can linger over the owner or stud for years.

Of course there are many excellent equine judges and they play a very important part in maintaining the enthusiasm and standards of care amongst horse ownership. But as in any walk of life, there can be one or two who let the side down with their manner or their comments, or even appearing to show unfair preference to a horse or an owner. One bias they can't be blamed for, however, is the impact of the wealthier owners who can afford the very best horses, but which then skew the odds for the other participants. So if you're 'just' a hobby shower it certainly pays to pick your shows carefully.

Mum also got involved which really pleased me. She wasn't keen on getting hands-on with the horses but she was very happy to do all the entry paperwork. And even when she was struggling with a respiratory illness towards the end she still liked to come along. We'd load her electric buggy and oxygen supply into the wagon, and once there she'd be in her element sitting by the ringside immersed in it all, telling anyone and everyone: *"That's my horse, you know!"*

To anyone who's never been to a show before it must look very strange and probably rather dull with all those people in the paddocks grooming and preening their horses. But for the owners it is just normal life, what they would do week in, week out if they could. I remember a lady chatting to me at a show about the hundreds of weekends she'd sacrificed to take her children and their ponies to shows. Then all of a sudden they left home and went away to university. *"Now I'm finding out what normal people do on Sundays,"* she said, *"and it doesn't involve standing in the middle of a muddy field in the driving rain!"*

But showing isn't just about the event day itself; the work starts long before. We had a horse, Lord Theodore, a beautiful liver chestnut we acquired who'd originally come to us for rehabilitation. He was a rig[28] and as a result a bit temperamental and sometimes stupid. However you just needed to show real

---

[28] A badly or incompletely castrated horse

determination with him, and he turned out to be one of our best show horses. But I had to spend hours tiring him out the day before or there was no way he'd behave on the day itself.

By 2005-6, however, things were getting out of hand. I was spending far too much time doing all the preparation and travelling to and from shows. I had a good team, but there was one member who had been pretty much pushed out of the picture altogether – Godfrey. He was supportive and very patient, but he had a life too and one that I was not making any time for. It wasn't just that he was becoming ever more immersed in politics; we had our own cricket club – the Horsehouse Formals – and to his credit the only time Godfrey was really angry was when I double-booked myself with shows and couldn't watch him play at Eton and in Ireland. He was absolutely right. To add insult to injury, Godfrey's company had been very generous by sponsoring classes and helping with the cost of equipment and sidesaddles. Mum's health was also deteriorating further, and so eventually and inevitably I just kind of hit the wall. All that adrenaline, that drive to win rosettes and trophies - I had become completely obsessed and I realized it had to stop. I had to find a different way to channel the competitive spirit and learn to spread my time more evenly.

If I had needed any further convincing, it would have been the simple economics of showing. When we first started and were just doing the local shows, the prize money just about covered the only significant expense, the cost of the diesel. But over the years prize money has dropped, entry fees have risen, and the whole enterprise has become very costly. So if you don't actually need the commercial boost that a win can bring to your stud, and you're not routinely selling horses, it becomes just a very expensive hobby.

I haven't given up completely on showing, but I've got it under control! I can say hand on heart that I don't actually miss the circuit at all, but I still attend a few shows each season that I sponsor, and enjoy them greatly. Also, my former assistant Kate convinced me to do just a little bit of showing - mainly low-key events where we've had great fun, emphasis on 'fun'. I've had some small highlights with a couple of horses - Mr Cracker who got through qualifying rounds for two successive years for Olympia's senior showing classes (and for the loan of which I owe much gratitude to my very good friend Mary Rook, who also generously lent him to Godfrey to ride too), and a nice maxi cob, Ted, a blue and white (who I still have and hope will become my next hunter) who won qualification at Osbaldeston in Lancashire for the Horse of the Year Show's 'Search for a Star' class. But anything remotely show-related nowadays comes a clear second to our other horse activities – and around the jaunts and outings that Godfrey and I enjoy so much.

And all those trophies? Well, it was always a thrill and an honour to win lovely antique silver trophies and statues with such a lot of history behind them. And as some of the shows no longer exist, their trophies reside in the attics of past show secretaries. But to restore the balance I have donated some new trophies of my own to a selection of shows – just a small way of giving something back to a world that gave me so much pleasure.

If you were ever a fan of the TV quiz show, Mastermind, you may
remember the time that Clare Balding, sports broadcaster, was in
the famous black leather chair. Her specialist topic was the Epsom
Derby; and one of the questions asked her to identify the jockey
who rode Portugese Lil to an unimpressive last place in the 1986
Derby. Why should this warrant a Mastermind question? The
reason was that the jockey, Alex Greaves, was the first female
jockey ever to ride in the Derby. But that's not all; Portugese Lil
was herself the first filly to run in the Derby – so a double first,
perhaps going some way to compensate for the dismal result.

Why am I telling you this? Well, in the 1990s, for a short time
after this famous race, I became the owner of this infamous horse.

I first encountered Portugese Lil, some time after her Derby race,
as one of my inpatients. I was treating her for sore shins, tilted
pelvis and torn hamstrings, and was due to send her back home
after twelve weeks of rehabilitation. However, home was with a
lady who looked after her for the owner who lived in Portugal;
and there was some muddle over money – she wasn't being
recompensed for my costs or something like that. Anyway, the
owner had either lost interest or lost the means to pay for her, so I
had the opportunity to buy Portugese Lil for a bargain price. And
that's exactly what I did.

My father had dabbled in horse racing in the 1970s, getting his
training license and having mixed success on the flat and over
fences, but I suspect he had more heartache from it than anything
else. So perhaps I had some trepidation myself as I took on this
racer, especially knowing the extent of her recent injuries. She was
a temperamental chestnut filly who tended to run her race before
she needed to and then ran out of steam too early, so I knew from
the outset that she was never going to be a winner; but I also felt
that that Derby race had been rather unfair to her. She was only

allowed to run because her father had himself been a Derby winner, and she found herself up against an entire field of testosterone-fuelled colts. Ironically this one very unequal Derby race then meant that she was given a hefty weight handicap in subsequent races, a great example of how ridiculous some of these racing decisions can be. I think her owner had only put her into the Derby so that he could brag about it. It was vanity really, not a decision made with the actual horse in mind, and had he not done so she might have been a more successful racer without this handicap.

Nevertheless, Portugese Lil gave me the chance to experience the sport of kings first hand for a season. Not a bad season either; between May and September, Lil ran in seven races, losing none of them and achieving fourth place in one. She continued to fight her jockeys, however, running her race too soon and fading away in the last furlong. In fact, she wasn't an easy horse at all and could be a bit of a witchy old cow to have around. But I think my real joy came not just from entering my own horse for races at Doncaster, Beverley and so on, but knowing that I'd made that horse sound after she'd first come to us completely broken. I went on to breed a couple of times from her, but both times she produced fillies with the same feisty and difficult temperaments, so I sold them on pretty quickly rather than getting embroiled in producing and training them myself.

Accompanied by Godfrey I had some great times at the races as a non-owner. Sometimes we were guests of large organisations at York, Beverley and Newmarket meetings, having a fabulous time in a box at the finishing line. Even more exciting were the occasions when Godfrey was himself entertaining his clients. I remember he once took a box at Wetherby and by the end of the afternoon he came out just a little ahead, having backed an outside odds horse called Yeoman Broker – a good choice given that he was entertaining insurance brokers. And at a Warwick meet I had the huge privilege of presenting the winning jockey, George Duffield, with a prize.

*

Competitive? Incapable of giving up? Stubborn? Whatever the reason, I've always been drawn to sports of many kinds, but looking back it seems that some of those that gave me the greatest pleasure were also the biggest disasters. I wonder what that's all about?

I've already talked about my school lacrosse – the one sport other than equine where I really shone (playing at cover point defence where on one occasion an opponent, a tough, unstoppable girl, came at me with such force that she broke my stick). My lacrosse prowess eventually waned when my rebellious phase overpowered my determination to succeed and I fell out with the captain of the first team. So let's see what else I got up to...

It was when I was working at Hull that I first took an interest in skiing, and I enjoyed several skiing holidays while still free and single. One in particular was an 18-30s holiday at Montgenevre in the French Alps. I had gone with a very good girlfriend of mine, Catherine, who shared my belief that the best skiing requires some strong liquid fortification.

I remember the fondue evening where huge quantities of alcohol were consumed – anyone who pulled their fork from the fondue without some meat on the end of it had to consume an alcoholic fine. The next morning I could hardly clamber on – and stay on – the button lift to the top of the slopes. Catherine wasn't much better. We were booked into a class to master some turn techniques (parallel and stem Christie). But it was all Catherine could do to stay in one place as she slid slowly down the slope with snow plough skis to the exasperation of the tutor who kept yelling: *"Parallelo, Catarina, parallelo!!"* – all to no effect as Catherine was wearing the thickest of ear muffs. Eventually she managed to come to a halt by skiing straight into the back of another lady in the class, which in turn sent us all toppling like a line of dominoes.

It has to be said that we were pretty determined to have a good time. Not for us waiting till the evening après-ski; we had après-lunch, usually consisting of *"deux grandes stellas s'il vous plait"* And duly refreshed we found our skiing had improved considerably, sending us confidently onto the red and black slopes. However, I remember one particular out-of-control moment when I was approaching a queue for the lift and found I couldn't stop. To avoid another domino incident I deftly swerved to the side and limboed my way smoothly under a fence and towards safety – one of my more elegant skiing moments!

Godfrey didn't share my enthusiasm for skiing: *"Why would I want to strap two planks of wood to my feet and hurl myself off the side of a mountain?"* So once we were married I was on the lookout for a suitable replacement activity. At college I had tried ice-skating, but having mastered the essentials – forward, turn and stop – I was soon on my backside with a broken wrist and no desire to continue. I had also previously dabbled in water skiing, again on holiday with a friend and again without much glory. On my first attempt I cautiously stood up on the skis as the boat accelerated, fell over backwards, got back up and then fell forwards with water shooting up my nose at 40mph. So I then tried replacing the skis with a board; this time I fell forwards, legs out flat, and bikini bottom flying through the air some fifty yards behind me.

To be honest I'd found water skiing a little scary – it was in the warm waters of Bahrain, filled with terrifying things like stingrays that I couldn't see from up above, and I felt very vulnerable treading water alone as I waited for the boat to turn round and pick me up again. So at the next opportunity I decided instead to try going beneath the surface - snorkeling. We were off Mombasa and it was all going unusually well; maybe at last I'd found my ideal water sport. Then someone came up in my blind spot and tapped my on the shoulder to point out some exotic fish. It scared me to death and I nearly drowned. And that did it for me. No more snorkeling; I'd be content with comfortable trips on the glass-bottomed boat.

179

Godfrey has an interesting theory for my series of sea-borne disasters; he says it is because half of my genes are from Poland, a land-locked country. And my Dad had always hated swimming ever since his days early in the war fighting with the German army; all the Polish recruits, renowned for being non-swimmers, were thrown in a canal on a sink or swim basis. So maybe Godfrey's theory is right...

Hunting has always been a huge part of my life, both before the ban and since, when hunting has been done by laying trails for the hounds to follow. So I can't tell my story without including it in the book; but, how do I do this while sidestepping controversy as much as possible? I realize that some people feel passionately about the topic and I'm not deaf to their arguments or closed to their feelings; I just wish perhaps that some of the more aggressive objectors might similarly open their own minds to a wider perspective. The popular image of hunting is often a myopic view of a very small minority that gives a lot of good people a bad reputation. However, for all readers, pro and anti, it wouldn't be fair if I didn't explain my own opinion a little first, and share what I suspect may be some lesser-known truths about the hunting community. So here goes.

Brought up in the muddy countryside with horses, a father who ran an abattoir and with farmers for neighbours, I learned about the harsh facts of life and death very early on. Mother Nature is cruel. Even so I include myself alongside the many people who have a strong instinct to save the lame ducks of the animal world. So I think for balance it is important to say that at least ninety percent of the hunting experience is about the ride and not the fox, something that the anti-brigade, peaceful or otherwise, doesn't always understand – and something I hope my anecdotes will bring to life.

Those who objected to fox hunting expressed two distinct frustrations in their campaigns - the social elitism of the hunt and the killing of the fox; and from my perspective it's not always clear which annoyed them the most. Certainly for anyone with a social chip on their shoulder the perception of 'snooty' hunting people makes the sport an easy target. But a demographic analysis of the average meet would show just how socially diverse and inclusive it can be. So that just leaves the fox element to be examined. Yet since the fox-hunting ban of 2004, hunts up and down the country do trail-hunting by law. Everything is the same as before except for one ingredient; the hounds are chasing a man-laid scent, not that of an animal. The idea, obviously, is that no animal should be hurt. But genuine accidents happen; rabbits, hares and foxes can suddenly pop up and run straight into the pack, although I've never witnessed this myself. And some saboteurs continue their aggressive tactics for distracting the hounds from the laid trail which paradoxically can lead them straight into the path of a fox!

So here's an interesting thought; if you could remove this small risk, and any unscrupulous illegal activity, and it was possible to trail hunt with complete certainty that there would be no accidents, then there would be nothing at all for anyone to object to. But I wonder, would that stop a load of people shouting abuse and calling us 'toffs'? And if not, would they also continue their own dangerous sport of blowing a horn to distract the hounds and lead them across busy roads, often to their deaths?

Hunting has also been used as a political football, to leverage advantage at Westminster and capture votes across the country. When an election is looming, for example, the Conservative Party knows that by promising a review of the ban in its manifesto it guarantees armies of free leaflet deliverers courtesy of the hunt members. And Tony Blair used the introduction of the ban to mollify his party's left-wingers who didn't like his Iraq policies. Meanwhile to the thousands of people who enjoy a day's riding cross country, it remains what it's always been, an equine sport.

One fact that cannot be challenged (although some still try) is that hunting provides invaluable rural employment. As with grouse shooting and other rural sporting activities, the hunts play a vital part in keeping the countryside alive and economically viable. Did you know, for example, that there is an organization, first set up in 1872 as the Hunt Servants Benevolent Society, that continues today to support the low-paid but often skilled people whose livelihoods depends on rural pursuits? It provides training opportunities and pension schemes, and it supports widows and others facing poverty. So, hunting reaches many layers of society and, I think, deserves to be better understood.

But that's me now climbing down from my soapbox. All I really want to do is tell you a few stories. Those familiar with hunting will easily recognise the scrapes I get into; and those not so familiar might enjoy a glimpse into a world where hoards of friendly people go out at least once a week in the coldest of weather for hours at a time, risking serious injury and at considerable expense. They can't all be mad?

*

Let's start by setting the scene. It's a cold Saturday mid-morning in February. The remains of an overnight frost still cling to the grass but the sun is just breaching the horizon. The hounds pace and jostle in a large scrum, whining in anticipation. The riders and their horses are assembling, tight columns of warm breath steaming from nostrils and mouths. However, much work has already taken place to reach this preliminary stage of the meet. In stables for miles around horses have been fed, mucked out and everything prepared for an evening return at the end of the day. Manes are plaited, horses tacked up, and there's just time to catch a quick cuppa before doing a Cinderella transformation from smelly stable clothes to best bib and tucker. I remember one embarrassing day when, creeping age having persuaded me finally to apply a little make-up before a hunt, I did so in the half-light of the stable. Once the hunt was underway, the bright midday sun revealed how heavy-handed I had been and I was destined to spend the day being alternately cheered and mocked for looking like Coco the Clown.

Preparation complete, at last you're ready to load up the horses and set off.

As you approach the meet, you have to find somewhere to park – a quiet lane nearby will do – and unload the horses, lock up the wagon, mount and set off. It's an electric atmosphere as the horses gather, the hounds already eagerly sniffing the air. But before the 'off' there is the essential therapeutic stirrup cup to enjoy, typically (but not always) comprising port or cherry brandy. With this there are usually a few speeches – welcoming visitors, commemorating recently deceased members and so on – and then the horn blows and the call rings around the crowd: "Hounds please!"

At this moment, good horsemanship and good manners go hand in hand. Riders must pull their horses back to let the hounds come through, and they must point their horses to the front so that they can clearly see the hounds around them; the last thing you want is for a hound to spook a horse and then receive a fatal kick from a hoof.

*

My earliest hunting memory is of falling off my horse. I was riding Gemini who had a penchant for bucking and rolling. He used to get hot and sweaty and, quick as a flash, would go down to roll in a puddle. The challenge for me was to see it coming and do a flying dismount to avoid ending up beneath him. Then when I graduated to jumping, he thought this was marvelous and would do extra big jumps that sent little me flying out of the saddle. On this occasion, down Yarmshire Lane at Knedlington, Gemini bucked me off into a large and deep puddle that completely submerged me. Fortunately Dad had the sense to give me the type of saddle with stirrup leathers that instantly disconnect – a safety feature allowing you to free you feet and leap to safety. Meanwhile the hunt followers tried to recapture Gemini, while I trundled behind, leathers in hand, very cross and swearing (and I remember being ticked off for that!)

After the hunt I would give Gemini a warm bran mash, some warm water to drink and a flap of hay before stabling him for the night with a sweat sheet and with fresh straw to dry him off. He'd spend one night like this and then be back out in the field for the rest of the week. I'm glad I learned this routine very young; it always saddens me a little to see how some people just pass their horse back to their grooms to sort out immediately after the hunt. I think when you've spent a whole day in the saddle (or mostly in the saddle in my case), you owe it to your horse to give it some personal attention.

Horses love hunting, of that there is no doubt whatsoever. But it can take its toll. A hunt can last just a couple of hours or, as often happened before the ban enforced trail hunting, it can go on for as long as there is daylight and a scent for the hounds to follow. This suited my brother who could be relentless once on the hunt. He used to hunt Charlie, and one day I'd got the horse ready for him – and off he went. We thought nothing more and expected him back by five at the latest when darkness would have fallen. Five came and went, and of course this being pre-mobile phone era, there was no way to find out if he was OK. We were growing really quite worried when he sauntered in just after seven with an exhausted looking Charlie. I was too worried about Charlie to be angry but it took nearly two full days for the horse to recover. He was just too tired to eat or drink, and only time, TLC and a lot of reassuring coaxing finally got him up and about again.

Above all, hunts are convivial affairs even if, once on the hoof, the assembly begins to disperse at different speeds (and sometimes, with errant horses, in different directions). And all good hunts start with the heart-warming Jumping Juice (the stirrup cup), but for some that isn't enough to sustain body and mind through a long, cold day in the saddle. One thing that Godfrey and my father had in common when out hunting was the careful provision of additional liquid refreshment for the day. Dad's preference was to fill his flask with vodka, and he was always very generous. If anyone showed an interest he was happy to offer them a swig

– but he never forewarned them that it wasn't hot sweet tea. You could almost see steam coming out of their ears as their eyes began to water.

I feel I have to say something about hunt saboteurs, if only because for so long they were an integral part of the experience of hunting.

By the early 1980s, saboteurs were hitting the Holderness hard (and sadly continue to do so). In my time I'd spent a lot of time with hound puppies, walking them as part of their training. They're lovely animals, and while anyone encountering the adults loose during a hunt might find them daunting the hounds are never remotely aggressive or pose any kind of threat. So there was one tactic to disrupt a hunt that I found especially unpleasant, not to say perplexing. The saboteurs would blow their own horn to distract the hounds and to draw them across a busy road, knowing that the riders couldn't follow. They seemed unconcerned by the inevitable canine fatalities, nor it seems by the potential for car crashes either.

I readily admit that a small minority amongst hunters could behave badly when confronted by protestors, and I don't think they did anybody any favours. And I know that even now there are rumours of law-breaking and animal cruelty. But I also think the level of acrimony and sometimes ignorance shown by the anti-hunt lobby is often overlooked. Personally I have no problem at all with people being able to express opinions; I believe in a libertarian society. But I think it must be done peacefully and with some basic courtesy and regard for others and for the landowner.

Country folk on the whole are far more tolerant than they get credit for; they approach life as a necessary compromise, not a rigid ideal. There are plenty of farmers for example who have experienced minor damage to hedgerows from the hunts, but they don't call for a complete ban because they understand the commercial value to the rural communities. They also live with, work with and respect animals. They would never, ever lead an animal into a potential death situation on a busy road, no matter how important their protest. So, looking back, I suppose there are lessons on both sides to learn from, but it has perhaps always been more difficult for the hunting fraternity to be fairly heard and judged.

Finally, even without foxes being killed, there are still casualties. Horse, hounds and sometimes riders can get hurt – it's a high-pace activity for people who relish a challenge, and things go wrong. But just occasionally it is something that could have happened anywhere, at any time. Many years ago we were out, once again on the Holderness Hunt, and word came down the line that a senior member of the hunt, Wilf Airey, had had a crashing fall from his horse. Those closest got to him very quickly but the poor man was stone dead. He'd had a heart attack in the saddle. There was tremendous sadness, but also the chance for some reflection. And I just wonder; for any man or beast that meets with an abrupt end while out hunting, is it such a terrible way to go - out with your chums in the bracing fresh winter air and sunshine, doing what you love so much?

*

I couldn't write this book without including one of my favourite poems by the perceptive and insightful Beatrice Holden, written before and during the Second World War. Many of her poems offer a poignant commentary on the changes experienced by the countryside and its dependents during the war. This one, however, beautifully articulates a problem that is as relevant to today's hunting riders as it was when she penned these lines.

Drop Your Hands

Tomm Firr indulged in a very big bit
(Always in pictures he's seen using it),
"Plenty of iron: you don't nee to use it."
"Yes, Firr – quite right, but *so many abuse it!*"

A light-mouthed pullers' a difficult horse,
A short-cheeked bridle will suit him, of course;
A snaffle the bit for a horse that takes hold
(At least, it's all right if the rider is bold).

The acme of bliss when you're hunting the fox
Is riding a horse who will jump off his hocks;
While quite the worst feeling, and one to be banned,
Is a horse which will only jump off his fore-hand.

"What *shall* I put on him, really I wonder?"
"Try to improve his ways with a 'secunder.'"
"Only unless you will ride for a fall,
I shouldn't get up on the beggar at all!"

All kinds of horses, all kinds of tackle –
Cut out the arguments, cut out the cackle;
A "bridle for scolds" I think should be found
For some of those writing for dear *Horse and Hound*!

Pelham or snaffle, Liverpool double?
What a commotion – what's all the trouble?
Dozens of letters from horse-loving lands –
It isn't the *bridle*, my boys; it's the *hands*!

By Beatrice Holden

From *They're Away*, published Collins 1945

You can find humour in almost anything if you look hard enough. And there's plenty of it in hunting, although most comes, rather painfully, from the inelegant moments when a rider is catapulted from their saddle to land somewhere in the mud below. One thing you can guarantee in life is that if you keep mounting horses, at some point you will come off. Here are just a few of my own high and low moments from hunting and other riding pursuits, all showing that if you don't take yourself too seriously, falls are (almost) fun and a good opportunity for some well-meaning mickey taking!

*

Dad and I first started hunting with the York and Ainsty South Hunt, but by the early 1980s were regulars with the Holderness when William Deakin was Huntsman. We had some marvellous days riding through lovely countryside ranging from the flat Holderness landscape to the slopes of the East Yorskhire Wolds. One less welcome feature of the Holderness, however, is the presence of huge ditches – land drains up to twelve feet deep and always a potential accident waiting to happen. Drains can appear relatively harmless until you're right up close and it's too late. I've had my share of falls and one drain that put the fear of God into me was Holderness's notorious Wigga Wagga.

You can get over a drain in two ways. One is simply to jump over it, but if it's too wide and the sides have a reasonable slope to them you can walk your horse down carefully to the bottom and climb back up the other side. Wigga Wagga was definitely one of the latter. I wasn't on Gemini this time but a rather dozy horse instead, and we'd made it safely to the bottom and were on the ascent when his back end gave way. As he slipped back down the drain I fired the ejector seat and landed on the bank. This startled him and he turned tail and legged it towards Hull.

Fortunately his progress was halted by another ditch where the banks weren't quite so steep, and I was able to catch up and grab his reins. But by now he had just become confused and stubborn and wouldn't budge. This is potentially very dangerous, particularly if the horse goes under the water as it gets cold and effectively gives up. Stuck like that for too long and horses can develop colic or chest problems. Some might even die. I was lucky, however – a knight in shining armour (Mr Ireland, a local farmer) was following the hunt, saw what happened and rescued us both. I've been back more recently over this patch of land and have seen how they now use mechanical diggers to create almost vertical walls to some the ditches. I'd definitely not take the risk of trying to cross those.

Falls are par for the course, but to have two in quick succession is sheer bad luck. I remember many years later hunting on a really feisty bitch, a chestnut mare I had bred. When she was on top form and really concentrating she could jump the moon, but at other times her jumping was very unreliable. It's the difference between a really good hunter and a so-so one; the best hunters can maintain a level head but the others just get too excited. The herd instinct kicks in, the adrenalin pumps and whatever you tell them they're just not listening!

The hounds were speaking and my horse was excited. We approached a fence and I had her perfectly lined up. Then something distracted her and she began looking to the side. I tried pressing all the right buttons but it was too late; she'd lost her focus and took off for the jump but failed to pick up all her legs properly. Bang! I was off. And so was she, buggering off at high speed but not before kicking me unkindly on the leg

As Dad had taught me, I got straight back onto my feet, and I took chase after my horse. Eventually, horse having been secured, we were off again and soon approaching another fence. This time I let go too soon and she hit the fence hard, launching me once again from the saddle. My brother, who was hunting with us, fortunately saw all this happen and came to my rescue. I'd felt a glancing blow from her hoof on my face, and could only see out of my left eye and feared the other one had been knocked out. I was assured it was just swollen shut. So we headed home, disgraced horse firmly to hand, and I was depatched to A&E where my nose and eye injuries were treated; no permanent damage but I had a rainbow bruise and couldn't open my right eye for several days.

And the horse? Well, Godfrey weighed in and forbad me from hunting her anymore. So off she went to another home that turned out to be the perfect match. Her new owner was a lad who liked to push her hard on the hunt and keep her in the thick of it. She simply didn't have the time or the energy to be feisty and argumentative.

Talking of Godfrey, he brought more than his fair share of comedic moments to the hunting field. First we had to match man and horse and we started Godfrey with Lord Theodore; not a great success as they were too alike – a little vain and easily losing concentration – so we tried Milo, the horse with no brakes. This was a much better partnership, Godfrey with a horse boasting a 'can-do' attitude with ears always pricked and eyes out on stalks, always up for it. This didn't stop him getting into trouble, however, one notable occasion being a New Year's Day meet with the York and Ainsty South. Godfrey and Milo were going far too fast and as they disappeared towards the horizon you could just see them overtaking the Field Master (a total breach of etiquette), with Godfrey shouting: *"Gangway Master...coming through!"*. The Master, Jeremy Timm, was extremely generous in forgiving this faux pas.

During the Lucy Glitters tour, Godfrey had joined us on The Percy, renowned for the Percy Special, their stirrup cup comprising a blend of whisky and cherry brandy. The hunt is also known for its generosity, so by the eleven o'clock departure we all had slightly spinning heads. We set off at our different paces and when I next saw Godfrey he'd stopped for a smoke and some more

Percy Special with a couple of other likely lads. I wanted to ride on so I left him partying and our paths next crossed an hour or so later. I was ready to pack it in for the day, but Godfrey appeared full of life – and with a suspiciously ruddy glow. *"Hello darling!"* he slurred to me from the saddle. Before I could reply, Milo, growing bored, turned a full circle, exposing the mud all over Godfrey's hat and a split in his coat from the waist up to the neck.

"Godfrey, you've fallen off haven't you?" He tried to deny it, but seeing I was about to lose patience he told me the whole story. There was a fence on a steep slope that I'd earlier decided was too dangerous to jump, choosing instead to open the gate and walk through. It turned out however that Godfrey had been unable to open the gate and so had decided there was no option but to jump. He and Milo took off superbly, apparently, but cleared the gate at slightly different moments; Milo had knocked the fence with a front leg and catapulted Godfrey before galloping off.

At this point in his story, Godfrey's face filled with pride: *"Listen darling, I got up and whistled like Roy Rogers calling Trigger – and bugger me if Milo didn't stop in his tracks and come back!"* I found this hard to believe, but as we retraced our steps we encountered some hunt followers who confirmed the story, and also told me what a superb jump it had been until the very last second. How could I stay angry with him after that?

Three of Godfrey's finer hunting moments were all during Middleton hunts. One day Godfrey was riding Mr Cracker and had been keeping company on the hoof with some pals – Roger Marley, Robert Tierney and Paul Smith come to mind – who all rode with generously filled hip flasks. Approaching a fence and with his judgement now unreliable, Godfrey rather feebly asked Mr Cracker to jump. Lacking a firmer instruction, Mr Cracker decided not to jump and came to an abrupt halt sending Godfrey sliding down the horse's neck and into the mud. *"What are you doing down there?"* Roger asked. *"Me? Oh I'm inspecting Cracker's hooves of course!"*

Another Middleton hunt, and this time Godfrey was riding Ruby, a great mare with a huge jump. He had been carefully instructed to trot her into the fences to encourage her to jump more economically. However, Godfrey thought better and decided instead to canter on approach - they jumped high and Godfrey fell out of the saddle and was knocked out. Fortunately Katie Stephens-Grandy and a couple of her lady chums were close by and tended to Godfrey who came to, surrounded by a bevy of beauties, and announced: *"I must have died and gone to Heaven!"*

And yet another Middleton hunt, one Monday morning: Godfrey rarely mixed politics and pleasure, but there was a period when he was in so much demand from the media that he had to have his mobile phone with him constantly. We were trail hunting by this time, and Godfrey had got himself double-booked, scheduled to appear on the Jeremy Vine radio show while in the saddle. So at the appointed time the two of us stopped on a hillside while Godfrey did his interview, and then resumed riding to try and catch up with the others. It had only been a few minutes but, unknown to us, a new trail had been laid that came right back towards where we were – and as the hounds came bounding towards us our presence completely confused the scent. This was a cardinal sin and we both got a huge bollocking from Peter McColgan who was in charge of the hounds. I remember we spent that evening writing humbling letters of apology and making appeasing phone calls.

*

I hope it's been enjoyable to read about what actually happens once the elegant throng has stopped posing in front of the country house and has dispersed along the field. To finish off, here are just a few more of my own memorable falls during hunting and other riding activities. Without becoming too serious, these remind us that any fall from a horse can be extremely dangerous. On the other hand, there's an old-fashioned saying that you need at least seven falls before you can consider yourself to be a serious horse rider...

One of the challenges when hunting is that you're riding with a lot of other people. So one moment you have a clear view of the field; the next all you can see is a horse's backside as you thunder towards it. This makes the accurate judging of hedges and other obstacles very difficult – as I found out one day at Birdsall near North Grimston.

I was riding 'No-Brakes' Milo, but all was going well. And I knew the land and calculated that we were approaching a particularly big hedge. As it came into view I watched as the rider ahead of me jumped it - and fell. I couldn't see exactly where he'd fallen and, not wanting to land Milo on top of him, I rode close to the hedge for a better look before taking off. It was too close and we jumped too late; over we went - and down we went, falling as if from a cliff. From this point on I have no recollection so I must have been concussed, but apparently I staggered to my feet and grabbed the reins, jumped straight back on and continued to ride – straight for another hedge, and splat. A double whammy – but this time I didn't let go and instead went skiing through the mud on my chest.

As this shows, concussion affects your judgement and makes you commit even more errors. The trouble is that by the time you are concussed it's too late to make rational decisions. And of course, it can happen any time you get on a horse, not just when hunting. One day I was schooling a young horse in the indoor arena. Godfrey was there too on his horse and we took it in turns to jump the hurdles. My young lad started being very cheeky and bucking on landing. At this point I should have made sure I sat tighter on the saddle, but I didn't, and he got me on the next jump. I have no recollection of what followed but it seems I got straight back on and continued to jump. Godfrey followed me over the jump and I then stopped and protested: *"Hey, when's my turn?"* I was clearly totally confused and had no idea what was going on. And the only memory I ever had of the incident was the splitting headache for two days with eyes that felt they were popping out of my had.

Finally, a fall without any concussion but one that instead extended the normal period of lost dignity by a full week. We were team chasing [29], and although it was in full view of my teammates my fall itself wasn't too embarrassing; but it did break my collarbone. The real problem was that in a week's time I was meant to be a decorative and helpful bridesmaid at a friend's wedding. And this was all I could think of as I lay in the mud in agony, hitting the ground with my whip and crying out: *"Oh f*ck!!"* To add to my shame, I'd only been working at Hull Royal Infirmary for one month and had not anticipated turning up as a patient quite so soon.

---

[29] A cross-country team race

"How nice it is to see Katie and friends adding prestige to any hunt, elegant ladies riding elegant horses [sidesaddle] so well. They covered our most testing country of hill, hedge and post and rail in their stride, the only downside being that they empty your hipflask, a small price to pay!" Joint Secretaries of the Middleton Hunt, 2004

If I had to declare any heroines, I would definitely include Lucy Glitters amongst them. Glamorous in a foxy kind of way, an actress and a skilled horsewoman and hunter - and entirely fictional - Lucy Glitters is the creation of the wonderful nineteenth century author, R.S. Surtees. Lucy eventually marries one of his best-known characters, the roguish not-quite-a-gentlemen, Mr Sponge ('Soapey' to his friends). Sponge is described by the R S Surtees Society as: "a horse-coper, the Victorian equivalent of a plausible and unscrupulous used-car salesman: he specialises in flogging spavined or ill-tempered nags, temporarily reconstituted, to credulous country gentlemen, and moving on to the next county before they realise what they have let themselves in for."[30]

Sponge worms his way into the hunting fraternity in search of a well-to-do bride, the Victorian hunting field being a prime place for a lady to meet a future husband. Side-saddle rider Lucy is not quite the wealthy heiress Sponge had hoped for but is desirable, described as *"tolerably virtuous"* and, most of all, a robust match for Sponge's unsentimental and opportunistic take on life. They set up their married home in Jermyn Street, St James's, London running Sponge's Cigar and Betting Rooms and tempting customers to *"indulge in one of Lucy's unrivalled cigars"* – until Sponge runs off alone to Australia in search of new adventures.

---

[30] http://www.rssurtees.com/product/our-commemorative-mr-sponges-sporting-tour/

Now, Surtees's story of this rogue is entitled: "Mr Sponge's Sporting Tour", so when I hit upon a ruse of my own involving a national tour of hunts riding sidesaddle, the perfect name sprang to mind: "The Lucy Glitters Sporting Tour".

But why sidesaddle?

I defy anyone not to have been impressed by seeing a well-presented sidesaddle rider, whether she was a lady out hunting or Her Majesty overseeing the Trooping of the Colour. The perfectly poised posture is eye-catching, and the outfit is extremely elegant. The most notable item is the habit; looking like a long coat it is in fact in three parts, a lighter coloured waistcoat, a jacket, and the apron which resembles a skirt but wraps around just the front of the rider. However, some details of the outfit vary depending on the nature and timing of the occasion. Autumn hunting and morning showing at county or royal shows require a tweed habit and a bowler hat; for the afternoon's final judging and for November hunting, this is exchanged for a black or blue habit and a silk hat. Beneath the habit is usually a white or cream shirt with a neatly tied dark tie. And finishing touches include neatly bunned hair to lift it clear of the collar, a cane in the right hand (to compensate for there being no leg on that side of the saddle) and for the ultimate in elegance a black veil can be worn.

But what about the poor old horse? Observers might easily think that having the rider all lopsided must be uncomfortable. And it's true; if the saddle isn't a perfect fit the horse will develop sores, and the lack of a rider's right leg can encourage the horse to become a bit crooked. But a correct saddle and some proper schooling in the normal astride seating position will counterbalance these problems.

Now, I'd already had some tremendous fun showing horses sidesaddle, and maybe it was dipping back into Surtees's novels that made me think of hunting sideways too – after all, how much more exhilarating to be riding in style across open countryside rather than just in the ring? And my chance came in February 2000.

An area branch of the Sidesaddle Association was having a special day with the Atherstone Hunt in Warwickshire. I decided to go, and I had the perfect horse, Maestro, a striking bay gelding built like a greyhound (a shire-thoroughbred cross), and originally my brother's horse that I bagged when he gave up hunting. Coming from local dealer Judi Thurloe, Maestro was a typically high quality horse although he could be a little scary – he didn't like queuing on the hunt, so once he had a fence or a hedge in his sight he locked on and went for it like an exocet missile; if anyone got in the way, we just had to jump over them.

The Atherstone meet was midweek on a cold and clear day, and there were about a dozen of us riding sidesaddle. However, with only a little experience of actually jumping sidesaddle, I was going in at the deep end and felt very apprehensive. I needn't have worried. In a lovely day of not too fast or furious riding with a good variety of terrain the worst that happened was almost losing my hat. Trevor Meeks, photographer for Horse and Hound, was capturing the drama of the event close up by lurking down low on the landing side of jumps; Maestro however spotted him and, anticipating a collision, put in an enormous leap which nearly launched me into the trees above, dislodging my hat. But it wouldn't have mattered to me if half my habit had been ripped off; after such an incredible day I was hooked. And back home that evening my mind suddenly exploded with an idea. I would compile an alphabetical list of hunts up and down the country, matching every letter from A to Z to a pack of hounds, and would work my way through each and every one of them, riding sidesaddle. The Lucy Glitters Sporting Tour was born.

*

The tour was to take four years to complete, concluding around the time of the 2004 fox-hunting ban. And I couldn't have done it without the support of all my staff or without Godfrey's sponsorship of this costly enterprise. I was also very lucky to have a team of horses ideally suited to this project. And so, with a banner made up for the windscreen of the horse wagon, I was ready to start. I just needed to work out the logistics of getting a group of horses and people to all these different hunts and locations:

A	Atherstone	N	North Northumberland
B	Belvoir, Duke of Beauforts	O	Oakley
C	Cottesmore	P	Percy
D	Derwent	Q	Quorn
E	Essex Farmers	R	Royal Artillery
F	Fernie	S	Sinnington
G	Goathland	T	Tynedale
H	Holderness	U	United
I	Isle of Wight	V	Vale of White Horse
J	Jedforest	W	Warwickshire
K	East Kent	X	Exmoor
L	Lincoln United	Y	York & Ainsty (N & S)
M	Middleton	Z	Zetland

The hunts closer to home could be picked off one by one, but for those further afield the only solution was to devise mini-tours to tick off a few at a time. Looking back they felt like world tours, such was the preparation required. However, Godfrey was an officer in the territorial army and recruited fellow officer Captain Mike Briggs who came to the rescue as a co-driver and logistics coordinator. And thus armed, we were ready.

Our first mini-tour took in Northamptonshire (the Oakley), Essex (East Essex Farmers), Wiltshire (Vale of White Horse) and Salisbury (Royal Artillery). Four days of hunting in a five-day programme – pretty busy and chaotic but wonderful fun. The Oakley gave us glorious sunshine and a couple of hours popping fences and chatting before boxing up and driving on to Essex and to our billet for the night. There everything had to be turned round, horses cleaned and the ones that hadn't hunted had to be exercised, but finally the humans got to relax over restorative drinks with the Hunt Master. Next day another good hunt, this time with the East Essex Farmers, and then on to Wiltshire, a very long drive after which we all just crashed out.

Godfrey had joined us at this point in the first mini tour, but it was a sombre occasion, the very last day of legal fox hunting (18 February 2004). The meet was also to be the final one for the Vale of White Horse Huntsman, and the after-hunting party was more like a wake, with people quietly ruminating on a lost way of life. The meet itself, however, was very hospitable; the stirrup cup on this occasion was gin and ginger wine – delicious. I'm sure I had more than I should have done, but soon we were off having first been told very clearly that there were to be two Hunt Masters, one for the more capable riders who wished to jump, and the other for the non-jumpers; we were to choose which to follow, based on our abilities, and stick to him. So at that point, Godfrey and I went our separate ways.

Fuelled by the Jumping Juice, and cheered by those who knew us with the call, *"Go Middleton Girls!"* we had a great time sailing over numerous hedges. Then, after about an hour and a half, there was a lull during which Godfrey caught up with us. Looking particularly flushed he announced with glee that he had jumped all kinds of things, despite being with the non-jumping party. He'd decided unliterally to interpret the instructions as more advisory than compulsory, permitting the occasional fence or hedge. Typical of Godfrey; I was secretly very proud of him.

We then had a free day before our meet with the Royal Artillery – a chance to clean all the tack, clothes and boots and generally get shipshape once again. It was to be another peculiar day. With the ban now enforced, no one quite knew what we were to do, but we still had a most enjoyable time in stunning open scenery with plenty of jumping. Signs of tiredness, however, were beginning to show. Godfrey had been riding Milo who was rather keen. Cantering up a long hill, Milo had suddenly stopped trying to pull and had adopted a more sedate pace, resisting all Godfrey's attempts to urge him on. We had to admit that humans and horses alike needed a rest, so after an early night we travelled slowly home for a period of recovery – and preparation for the next mini-tour.

*

This time we were to start by crossing the waves to join the Isle of Wight meet. We were greeted by yet another gloriously sunny and frosty morning – but now with rolling downs on the northern side of the island and dramatic drops down to the sea. Milo was back on top form, pulling as hard as ever with a very worried Godfrey in the saddle assessing the proximity of the sheer drops. At least I knew I had my husband well insured. But we had a good day without accidents, made even better by meeting up with an old friend, Richard Standing, who had been a whipper-in[31] many years earlier with the Holderness and was now here as Huntsman.

The following day Godfrey had to leave to get back to London so I took the horses on myself from Southampton to Exmoor. I remember it being a hair-raising drive up and down extremely narrow and twisting roads, but I eventually reached my destination for the night, the Crown Inn, Exford, in good time to settle the horses. The next day was free and while I was exercising them I noticed a definite feel in the air – there was a bad cold snap on the way. And by dusk snow was falling. Things weren't looking good for the hunt.

Sure enough the next morning the ground was covered with a white icy carpet and the hunt was cancelled. But the Masters and Huntsmen were heroes and rose to the occasion. They insisted that we still get togged up in our sidesaddle gear, and then,

---

[31] A person who keeps the hounds in a hunt organized and focused while out in the field.

somewhat gingerly, we mounted the horses for a photo shoot with the hounds. It was the only hunt on our A to Z that didn't actually happen, but I felt our combined efforts warranted it being ticked off the list. Needless to say, the next day as we prepared to set of home there was no sign of snow at all.

I can't go through every hunt with you – and it would become very dull indeed if I did. But there are just a few more happy memories worth sharing, starting with the Belvoir. Run from Waltham in the Wolds, the Belvoir has some of the biggest hedges I have ever jumped; it also has the members with the keenest sense of their own importance. And in their hands there were some particularly feisty horses that were in danger of jumping on the hounds. I am always angry to see the welfare of the hounds being overlooked, and felt obliged to tell the thrusters[32] to hold hard, to which a couple retorted: *"WE are the Belvoir and WE will do what WE like!"* What rudeness and what disregard for animals! They would never have got away with that at the Middleton; Frank Houghton Brown, Master and Hunstman, would probably have tried to kill anyone who threatened one of his hounds.

One hunt that sticks in my mind for all the wrong reasons is the Sinnington which incorporated breakfast, a gallop and then a days hunting. After a few glasses of champagne with breakfast we set off on the gallop, and I was so lucky to be escorted and tutored over the fences by our host, Mary Holt, a superb sidesaddle rider. All was going well until we came to a small jump next to a five-bar gate that was slightly ajar. As shown by Mary, I approached on a really good stride when my horse suddenly veered left away from the jump and towards the gate. It was too late to stop, so I kicked hard and he took off but snagged the gate, bringing part of it with us. I shot off like a catapulted stone, but still holding on to the reins. Fortunately the horse ground to a halt – and, even more fortunately, there was a doctor on the gallop who came to check

---

[32] The term for riders who ride too close to the staff or hounds

me over. I was fine, just bruised pride, but I can't say the same for the doctor; clearly unfamiliar with the sidesaddle outfit and trying to retrieve the apron of my habit he accidentally gave me a jolly good groping.

And there were many other memories that stick with me: joining the Middleton in the presence of Prince William and his chums – I was able to shine, flying over the big hedges, having been tipped the wink by Field Master Simon Roberts so that I didn't get sucked into the melee of stoppers and fallers; the day with the United in the Welsh Borders where, caught short, I dismounted and bobbed down in a secluded place only to see a row of hunt followers in their cars all watching in amazement – no doubt intrigued to see how a woman managed a pee when done up in the habit; and the Goathland, memorable for less than honorable reasons – it's a farmer's pack, no pretensions, and having already been riled by the flamboyant arrival of a follower in a helicopter, they couldn't resist the opportunity to have a bit of mischief with the snooty Middleton ladies who had been invited to the meet by leading us onto the boggy moor.

*

At the time of the Lucy Glitters tour, sidesaddle hunting was still a rarity but I'm delighted to see how it's popularity has grown since – and it would be lovely to think we helped that to happen. But let me finish with a caveat to anyone who may be inspired to take up sidesaddle hunting for the first time – you need to be exceptionally fit! To sit at that sideways angle and have complete control of the horse for three or four hours of hunting requires strong abdominals and good core strength. If you don't do your preparatory fitness regime, you may find you looking for a sympathetic physiotherapist...

"Does Katie Bloom live up to the stereotype expected of a UKIP[33] wife? All twinset and pearls, received pronunciation and cucumber sandwiches?" So begins a feature on me in the Daily Mail from August 2013, examining what it's like to be the wife of one of UKIP's then most notorious figures.

It's a cleverly constructed article, opening with a proposal that will soon be cunningly contradicted to whet the reader's intrigue. But it still requires two more sentences to set up the big surprise: *"The wife of Godfrey Bloom, the UKIP MEP, is rarely photographed with him and appears to play no part in his political life. Perhaps she is shy and fragile, living in the shadow of her ebullient husband?"*

And then, perfectly timed, comes the revelation: *"Mrs Bloom strides up to greet me warmly in a thick Yorkshire accent, wearing jeans and a polo shirt. It's fair to say that she probably does not conform to most people's idea of a UKIP wife. Indeed, she reveals that her husband calls her his Commander-in-Chief. At home, it is Mrs Bloom who is in charge."*

However, there are a couple of things that puzzle me about this piece of journalism; firstly the interviewer insisted that I have a full make-over and hair do and put on a posh frock for the photo shoot. It was great fun, but not really true to the image she was trying to portray in the text; and secondly, she wrote mostly about Godfrey's political reputation rather than his married life. This in itself didn't bother me, but there is always more to find out if you ask the right questions, and Godfrey is certainly much more than 'just' a UKIP man.

---

[33] United Kingdom Independence Party

I couldn't write this book without giving a special place to Godfrey, so I hope this chapter will plug a few of the gaps left by the article and reveal a little more about the man I chose (eventually) to marry and have lived happily with for over thirty years.

*

To me, Godfrey is all about life, loyalty and love. And in thirty-one amazing years of marriage we have developed a double act that works extremely well because of two ingredients – our shared interests and our shared capacity to support each other's endeavours. Never one to crave the limelight, I was happy not to stick myself at the centre of his political life, but did and will always stand solidly by him when required, And it works the other way too; being husband to a workaholic equine fanatic will not have been easy, but Godfrey has always been there, helping make sure I can stand on my own two feet and achieve what even I sometimes think is out of reach.

To explain how our relationship works would be impossible unless you were to join us in front of a log fire for a lazy evening, an excellent whisky in hand as we digest a delicious lamb curry, or at breakfast when I'm coming back from early horse chores to the best bacon buttie you've ever tasted (both meals expertly cooked by a daintily-aproned Godfrey). So instead I'll share some memories and anecdotes.

Godfrey and Katie – The Major and Mrs B as we tend to refer to each other – very nearly didn't happen. Twice.

The first time I met Godfrey was in 1984 at a hunt ball: *"Hello, my name is Godfrey,"* he announced, slurring his words. *"I'm extraordinarily rich you know; so would you like to dance with me?"* Unimpressed I turned him down flat. And that was that for more than a year, until our paths crossed once more. This time he moderated his approach, I decided to give him a second chance and we began to get acquainted. And within a few months we were married. But not before Godfrey safely crossed the second hurdle...

Godfrey respects tradition, so having proposed to me in November 1985 at the Badsworth Hunt Ball in Scarborough's Royal Hotel, he decided to ask for my father's approval. He was already more than a little in awe of Dad having learned of his ruthless wartime survival experiences, so this was no small undertaking. And what if Dad had said no? Anyway, the following Sunday Godfrey came to lunch early, intending to speak to my father before the meal. He stopped the car outside the Vicarage paddock gate, left the engine running in case a hasty retreat was called for, and walked nervously towards the yard. Meanwhile, to discourage any sudden *volte face*, I cut off Godfrey's escape route by patrolling the entrance with a laden wheelbarrow.

Unusually for an eager talker, Godfrey struggled to find his words. His cop-out opening line: *"I guess you know why I'm here?"* was met with complete silence, so he had to bite the bullet and articulate his question clearly. Dad remained silent, and Godfrey immediately began to backtrack: *"Of course, if it's no dice just say the word; we can scrap the whole thing, kick it into touch, right under the carpet, least said soonest mended...."* Dad turned, still silent, and walked indoors. Glancing in my direction, Godfrey gestured as if to ask: *"is he getting his shot gun?"* But no, it was just lunchtime, that was all. So, having switched off the car, we followed him in and joined the family at the table for a meal that drowned in awkward silences and pauses. Godfrey swears that he caught Dad glancing up at the gun cabinet several times during lunch, but in the end approval was granted.

One of the many of Godfrey's qualities that I admire is his pragmatic approach to problems and opportunities. He is not one to sit on the sidelines tolerating incompetence if there is a way to make things happen more efficiently (or to put it another way, he calls the proverbial spade exactly what it is). You might even conclude that this is a genetic feature of the Bloom bloodline and something that has been ably demonstrated in the field of military service. Godfrey's father, Alan, had been an RAF Spitfire pilot in World War Two, surviving the war but sustaining burns to his hands and face on HMS Furious when it was configured as an aircraft carrier. And his mother, Phyllis also looked to the skies as a sergeant in the Women's Auxiliary Air Force.

Godfrey's own soldiering was more down to earth, clocking some thirty successful and colourful years in the Territorial Army, and ending up as head of recruitment and training for a Yorkshire Territorial Regiment. But as Godfrey's two sisters proved, the Bloom flair for competence hasn't been restricted to the armed services. Margaret, the eldest and now sadly deceased, played a mysterious and shadowy role in the secret service; and Hilary, the younger sister and now retired, was herself a very able and accomplished personal assistant. I think for Godfrey, however, the TA was more than just about the military; it provided an outlet for some of his other innate skills, in particular working with human nature. And of course, it also offered ample social opportunities too...

Godfrey is definitely a party animal and, despite his best efforts, a combination of beer and mischievous chums has often led him into a spot of bother. Whilst always perfectly harmless, this has sometimes been an inconvenience to me as his wife but is also such an endearing side to his character that I always have to forgive him. Once, early in our marriage, I took him to our local pub, The Barnes Wallis, for a pre-dinner drink. After a considerable time I was anxious to get home and finish off the cooking. But Godfrey, his words beginning to slur, pleaded to stay for just one more pint – and then promptly fell over. The pub's clientele broke into cheers and applauded as he awkwardly hauled himself back upright and, quick as a flash, declared: *"Damn. I think that's scuppered my chances of one for the road!"* I could barely keep a straight face.

Did I say *"I always have to forgive him?"* Maybe that's not strictly correct, not unless forgiving comes with a small price-tag attached.

You see my husband embraces life in the moment, and I love this about him even if it means a spontaneous U-turn from what had been planned. But when it is me who is left hanging, we have grown accustomed to using a system of fines; and it is I who decide on the size and nature of the fine. I'm sure Godfrey agrees that this works really well, leveling the playing field and preventing any lingering ill feeling. Here are just a couple of examples.

Godfrey had been working in London but was due back later that evening. I remember it was shortly after the IRA had bombed the Carlton Club, so I was never really relaxed until he was safely home. He rang me to say he would be on the York train leaving King's Cross at eight in the evening. So I decided to drive to York and surprise him at the station. Standing alone on the chilly dark platform, I watched the train come to a halt and the passengers disembark. No Godfrey. And of course this was before mobile phones, so I couldn't call him.

I did try phoning his club, however, and left a message but he can't have got it as, the next morning, he phoned me to explain that his train had been cancelled. It was only when I told him that I had watched that same 'cancelled' train arrive and depart that he came clean – he'd been drinking with city friends, missed the train and crashed on someone's sofa. When he finally turned up, in time for a family Sunday lunch that I was cooking, he volunteered: *"Don't worry Mrs B, I'll put myself in the dog house..."* referring to the utility room where our dogs sleep. But I had a better idea. I would impose one of my fines, this time a lovely dress from Droopy and Brown to go with other similarly extorted items in my wardrobe.

You would think that a gregarious man so prone to the temptations of socializing would learn a few tricks; but no, not Godfrey. If anything he got worse at trying to cover his tracks. I remember one instance of this when he had started to work in Brussels as an MEP. The journey home now involved not one but several train journeys, each of which could 'go wrong'. One day Godfrey called me on the mobile to say he was stuck in Brussels traffic on the way to the station and it looked likely that he'd miss the last channel tunnel train. And sure enough, I could hear traffic in the background. But I could also hear laughter and then a voice calling out: *"Are you having another beer, Godfrey?"* I was so angry; I remember putting the phone down on him and deciding there and then that the fine this time would be an expensive new sidesaddle.

*

When two people have to spend days at a time apart as we did, it's always helpful to have some common interests to reset the relationship glue; and ours included horses and hunting. However, this was another aspect of our life that nearly didn't happen.

Godfrey had learned to ride a few years before we met at Joyce Fern's riding school in Beverley and had enjoyed some hacks on the Beverley Westwood. He even took himself off once to the Lake District on a Dales Ponies riding holiday; apparently he fancied the girl who owned the ponies. However, when we began dating, my Dad nearly extinguished Godfrey's interest in riding for good. The three of us used to go riding together with no problem, but one day Dad took Godfrey out without me; and he took the opportunity to pull Godfrey down a peg or two by giving him a frisky horse and then, by playing up the danger, convincing him to lead the horse back through the village on foot – very humiliating. It actually shook Godfrey's confidence in riding and he only really took it up again some fifteen years later in 2004. I had persuaded him to book a holiday for us in Argentina – and it just 'happened' to include riding. He struck a deal with me; if he enjoyed his South American riding, he would agree to spend one day hunting with me back home and see if it grabbed him. Fortunately it did, and our great riding adventures began.

You will have discovered some of Godfrey's hunting capers in an earlier chapter. And certainly, hunting was in many ways the perfect sport for such a social animal – not just fresh air and exercise wrapped up in convivial company but the only sport that positively encourages a stiff drink before midday. We did, however, also continue to enjoy the occasional ride when on holiday, and one year even booked a short riding vacation, USA-style. Needless to say, it would not go completely smoothly...

We had been due to visit some friends in America, and decided to go over a little early and experience something new - ranch riding in Wyoming. We stayed at Paradise Ranch near Buffalo; and having gone through a careful vetting process to assess our riding abilities when we made the booking, we awoke the first morning eager to see what horses we'd be allocated.

Godfrey, classed as a beginner, was given Clint, a reliable horse who looked after him admirably; I on the other hand had been listed as experienced and "don't really mind what I ride..." and ended up with a pottery horse that was clearly footsore and stumbly at the front end. I could help him along by hooking him up in his mouth, but it wasn't much fun for the poor old horse who nearly fell on his nose at one point while taking a lame step. I decided he was definitely not fit for riding and I would say so the next day if asked to ride him again.

Sure enough, the following morning, out came Clint and my poor old soldier, so I said *'no, absolutely not'*. The other riders on the parade ground watched in silence as the organisers huffed and puffed at me; but I held my ground. The horse was lame, I said, and should not be ridden. No response; it seemed they didn't like being told. So Godfrey came up alongside me: *"My wife is a leading equine physiotherapist; and if she says that horse is lame, then it's lame."* My hero. After a further lingering silence, a replacement horse was eventually brought out.

However, as we rode away I glanced back to see a groom on the lame horse, kicking and whipping it and hooking it in its mouth to stop it from falling. This is terrible treatment, a brutal and unforgiveable 'quick fix' to make a horse take particular care. And we heard that later that week someone had come off a horse that had stumbled badly...

More recently Godfrey has had to give up riding altogether after some back surgery, which is a great sadness to us both. But it's given us an excuse to devote more time to another great love of ours, walking holidays. And there's a nice symmetry to this too, as our first holiday together, before we were married, was spent fell-walking near Keswick. We each took a friend with us, and I remember Godfrey's chum having us in stitches as he tried and failed to get his tent pegs into the ground; meanwhile Godfrey monkeyed around, stuffing entire chocolate digestives into his mouth. But it was the beautiful walks that stay with us the most. And we decided to honeymoon in the Lake District, walking every day after a hearty breakfast and returning just in time for a soothing bath and a gourmet dinner. Since then I think we've covered pretty much all of the Lakes, with friends or on our own with our dogs. Crumbling joints eventually led to a cessation but, following hip and knee replacements, we're back on the trails once more – although these days we tend to stick to the slightly easier Dales and coastal paths.

*

Well, I've got through a very long chapter with barely a reference to politics! But of course, Godfrey's time as an MEP did impact on me and on our life together, so I can't finish without just touching on the actual business of being the wife of a politician, and of a controversial one at that...

From the antics I've shared about him, it's obvious that Godfrey would hit the world of politics with a bang (or should that be a bong(o)?) No quiet back-benching for him. His interest had been growing for some time. Many hours were spent in the pub with chums who all moaned about the state of the country whilst offering nothing more useful than a resigned "Well, what can you do, eh?" And Godfrey, growing more and more frustrated by this apparent impotence, finally decided he wanted to see what, if anything, could in fact be done; his intention was to give his very best and, if nothing came from it, at least he had tried, unlike the public house moaners' chorus. So, in 2004 he stood for the European Parliament as a UKIP member and was elected - and thus I became a politician's wife, and was quietly very proud of Godfrey for stepping in and having a go.

Ten years of some very mixed experiences followed – from gangs of photographers camping on the doorstep to the chance to travel to some amazing places such as India and Morocco. But during this time it's been rare that Godfrey has actually needed a politician's wife on his arm; I've been there more as the companion who would have been there anyway, whatever he'd been up to.

Those doorstep reporters were at their most invasive when Godfrey's "Bongo Bongo" comments were in the news, back in 2013. And it wasn't just our doorstep; they were swarming all around Wressle looking for comments and quotes from the other villagers - and not just about politics, but anything that they could use to discredit Godfrey. We were amazed and touched by how supportive everyone was, telling them in polite or not-so-polite terms to clear off and leave him alone. "*He's a friend of ours!*" they said again and again. One eager reporter unwisely knocked on the door of a house belonging to a wonderfully diffident resident. She hardly ever used her front door, and so appeared from the side of the house to reprimand the reporter: "*Stop knocking on the door – you're upsetting the cats!*" Undeterred, the reporter began to fire questions. Her reply, as she walked away, cat under her arm, summed up what most people felt: "*Why would I care...?*"

Journalists have to be tenacious; it's part of the job description. And so, having exhausted Wressle they moved on to Howden, targeting the shops and pubs where Godfrey drinks. However, knowing and admiring Godfrey as they did, none of the traders, shopkeepers and landlords would say anything and so, as a last resort, the hacks tried Rotherham. There they found some inarticulate people and reframed their questions to elicit some negative comment. But seriously, they may as well have gone to Southampton and interviewed a schoolchild who had never heard of Godfrey; it was hardly the scoop they'd been looking for!

We did, however, discover for ourselves that even if you can shake off the journalists, you can't so easily disassociate yourself from the political identity; there's no 'down time'. This struck me the most on off-duty occasions when we were just mooching around on our own as we've always done, going to events, wandering in and sitting quietly at the back, seeing what's going on. At the height of UKIP's media attention we had to wave goodbye to this causal anonymity; as soon as we sat down, flustered hosts or organisers would scurry up to us uttering all kinds of groveling apologies and hustle us up to the front to join the other 'prominents' in the special reserved seats. This kind of experience left very mixed feelings – a little pleased to be given special treatment, annoyed not to be allowed to remain invisible at the back, and not a little p*ssed off to be exploited as some kind of status symbol for the event.

The political world was fun, challenging and sometimes frustrating – but really it was Godfrey's world and his job; I had more than enough of my own to deal with. And today, while Godfrey continues to be in demand as a Libertarian speaker and an independent commentator on the unfolding Brexit process, the man who still calls a spade a spade, for the rest of our time we enjoy being simply The Major and Mrs B once more, a sociable double act that works just fine for us and our friends. And cheers to that!

I had the great privilege to help Katie write her book. And as with any good autobiography, it is not just the retrospective telling of a story but a journey of discovery. Katie's journey, of course, is far from over – barely even beginning to slow down – and that creates a problem for an editor; how do you wind up a book when the story is still going strong?

The easiest trick is to talk about 'bucket lists', all those ambitions and dreams that she might yet fulfill. But sitting down with Katie to talk about this, it became clear that for her, and also for Godfrey, the bucket is pretty empty. And this is not surprising – they have pursued their lives together energetically and pragmatically. When something has caught their interest, they have gone after it with focus and purpose, driven by an appetite for new experiences; not for them jotting down an idea, putting it in the hypothetical bucket and hoping to get round to it before it's too late.

I don't, however, think their attitude to life is any way reckless or gung-ho. Quite the opposite in fact, and the Lucy Glitters Tour is just one testimony to the depth of detailed planning that has underlain so many of their adventures. And this is what has struck me most about Katie's story – her ability to take impressive risks while simultaneously keeping her feet firmly on the ground.

So, I hope the unusual blend of life story and special interest has worked. However, it struck me that whilst Katie's life has revolved around horses, it might just have easily have been pigeon racing or investment banking – the underlying storyline would still be that of a modest but rather remarkable half-Polish, half-Yorkshire lass 'made good'. And I wanted to return one last time to this as a way of rounding off the book. So I decided that the best way to pin down and distil some of Katie's innate qualities was through an interview. Katie agreed, and it went something like this…

*

Katie, I'm certain that you will strike your readers as a quietly industrious person, not a fame-seeker. So I'm curious why you agreed to write and publish your own story?

Well as you know it was originally Godfrey's idea. And when he first raised it my initial thought was simply that I wouldn't have time! But he persisted and encouraged me to begin thinking about my life and my work, and I realized that I have been lucky to live quite an interesting life. However, I think I share my husband's need to speak out or take action if something needs to be said or done; and I also firmly believe that hard work really is its own reward, something the younger generations have lost touch with. So if my story helps in some way, maybe to improve general horse care or encourage people to knuckle down and pursue their dreams, then it was worth writing.

And have you enjoyed writing the book?

Ah, well yes, but it's been tough! Not just the hours it takes, but having to revisit old half-forgotten memories, some good, some bad. There were nights when I was almost in tears, it all churned up so much from my past. But yes, it's like any project, exciting to take the first step and just as exciting to see it all finally come together.

Neither of you take yourselves too seriously; but you have both clearly achieved a great deal in your life. What do you think for you, Katie, are your greatest accomplishments?

Well, my life's not over yet! But I think in some ways I've been lucky in my timing; in both the human and equine work I was training or honing my skills when the professions were still evolving. With human physiotherapy, I qualified at the time when it was first becoming a more widely accepted and respected part of the medical team and toolbox. And the equine work was in a way right at the start, when the profession first gained a formal and approved status.

It's always exciting and motivating to be in at this stage. There's a kind of dynamism and, I don't know, an intrepid energy. There weren't many rulebooks or comprehensive textbooks, so you had to use your brain and your common sense and to some extent feel your way. It's something I really feel is wrong nowadays. A young professional today in the health service has to conform to so many rules and health and safety instructions, they must feel so restricted when it comes to developing their professional instinct; and to be honest, I'm not sure people today are taught any more to use their brains anyway.

Sorry I'm rambling; so, what have I achieved? Well, I guess I looked for opportunities rather than waiting for them to find me, I seized them, put in the hard graft, learned my trade and always went that little bit further, not taking dangerous risks but daring to try something or to say something that could make a difference even if it goes against the perceived rules.

Do you think rules are there to be broken then?

That depends. When you're young, yes, you should have the chance to challenge the rules – and to face the consequences; it's part of growing up. But no, rules are important as a framework; but they must be sensible ones, not just there for the sake of it. There are so many organisations that start off with great ideas or intentions, and then become so laden with bureaucracy, rules and sub-committees that they almost cease to function. I'm all for freedom, and sometimes you need rules to protect that; but when the rules get in the way, then something's gone wrong.

OK – now, not the most imaginative question but here goes; who or what do you think has had the biggest influence in how you've approached life and work?

That's an easy one; it's my father. We live in interesting times when immigration has come to mean different things to different people. But back then, just after the Second World War, immigrants were definitely welcome. And the difference was that anyone coming new to the country wanted to work and work hard; not just that – they wanted to fit in and in effect become English. My Dad was no different, and his story shows just how hard-working he was; and I think that was the strongest influence on me.

Was your father proud of his Polish roots?

Oh yes, but that's not really the point. What mattered was what other people thought; they saw him working all hours, running successful businesses. And they saw him making the effort to get involved and integrate. He earned their respect. These days I'm not sure all newcomers to the country try so hard. Or perhaps we just don't expect them to. In fact there are a couple of stories I can tell you that show how different things are today and how appalled Dad would be if he was still alive.

My brother's daughter (and she was born and bred in Yorkshire) recently had to be admitted to hospital towards the end of her pregnancy. Now, she still has the Polish surname, Skowronek, and the nurses assumed she was a health tourist, here to make use of the NHS, and treated her disrespectfully. Meanwhile, there were some ward cleaning staff from Poland who spoke to her in Polish, automatically assuming she was over here temporarily to earn money. To my father these would have been unforgiveable assumptions. But he would probably have come down hardest on the new generation of immigrant workers who don't make the effort to integrate. My brother, for example, has a young Polish lad working for him whose spoken English improves noticeably during the week, but then, after the weekend, has slipped back to pigeon English. And the reason? He spends his weekends exclusively with other Polish people, even going to a Polish-speaking church.

So, no, we in our family are all proud of our Polish heritage, but just as proud of being English, and especially from Yorkshire. In fact, when someone challenged my brother for having a foreign surname (Skowronek) he had a brilliant reply – "Nonsense, it's a very old Yorkshire name – in fact it goes back as far as the 1940s."

Wonderful stories, thank you – but I'd like to get back to you. If you could turn the clock back, is there anything you would do differently?

Are you asking about regrets? I don't really have those. I haven't got time for them! But let me think. I suppose I would try to pace myself better. I can be impulsive and, once I see a goal, I tend to go for it with all I've got. Sometimes it's better to be more patient and circumspect. I'd also try – but I wouldn't make any promises – to keep my trap shut rather more often. I've always told it how it is, regardless of whether it'll do me any good or not. Maybe it's all part of the blunt Yorkshire honesty?

Dad had a phrase that I could perhaps have remembered more often – "Every day is a holiday!" And when I think back to my early working years, I was like many young, ambitious people, driven by having no money and a fear of failure. But since then I've been so lucky to be working in something I love that I've grown to appreciate each and every day, even dark, cold Monday mornings. And that's probably the only piece of advice I'd give to today's youngsters – never forget what a privilege it is just to be here, and always try to make the most of it – and enjoy it.

Can I ask you to look forwards this time, and tell me what you see in the future for your profession, specifically the equine work?

Well, like any medical speciality, it goes in peaks and troughs, but I think it faces an uncertain future. So much has changed since I first began working with horses. Let me give you an idea. I had to work really hard to build up my reputation; and part of that process was to earn the trust of the local vets so that they felt comfortable prescribing my service, happy to leave me to work out exactly what was needed. And of course that relationship of trust was critical if, between us, we were to treat horses promptly and correctly.

Since then two things have changed it all. One is the growing influence of insurance; take a sick horse to a vet and the first question you're likely to be asked is whether or not it is insured. And your answer may, (but I only say may,) influence the suggested course of treatment (and who delivers it) if there is more money to made in insurance fees. This skews the professional relationship and also the choices facing the owner.

The other big change of course has been technology. And I'm talking as much about simple things like bandages as about complex computerized instruments. A modern dressing can heal the kind of wounds that in the past would routinely have been referred to us to treat with lasers and so on. And this is great, but it does beg the question, what is the physiotherapist there for? And our profession has to keep getting the message out there - that our intuitive, hands-on, individualized approach both to diagnosis and to treatment can never be entirely replaced by computers or smarter bandages. No two animals and their injuries are identical, and to my knowledge they have not yet invented the computer that can apply human experience and intuition to animal health.

That's fascinating, so presumably the professional association is working hard to clarify this?

I'm not 100% sure what ACPAT[34] is doing. It's actually one of those organisations I mentioned a moment ago that in my opinion lost sight of it real purpose and became more focused on its own internal functions. I actually made the very difficult decision to

---

[34] Association of Chartered Physiotherapists in Animal Therapy

leave ACPAT when I felt it was not looking after the interests of its members. A colleague of mine, an experienced physio of some twenty years of more, was hauled up by ACPAT for "practicing outside of their scope of expertise" after administering some aromatherapy to a pony. It was a messy story, but I felt it amounted to a betrayal of trust in the membership and I immediately resigned.

That must have been a very difficult decision to make?

Oh yes. I still have very mixed feelings about ACPAT. I mean it was a huge part of my professional life early on, and a great privilege not just to be a founder member but to work on its behalf, running conferences, lecturing, helping to set up the postgraduate RCVS course. But as I said, things go in peaks and troughs, and I am sure the association will recover its strengths and play its part in the future of the profession.

So who exactly is looking after the interests of new and would-be equine physiotherapists?

Well to be fair to ACPAT, there are some changes that even it can't protect its members from, particularly the self-employed ones. For example, we've seen more and more small veterinary practices being swallowed up by larger firms, and they employ their own therapist who covers an enormous patch. Also the profession still tends to be female-dominated, and as well as those wanting to leave in order, say, to raise a family, women are perhaps more likely to be doing it for vocational reasons rather than monetary reward. So as simple business pressures come to play, those people will inevitably fall away.

Now, if I was just starting out as a newly-qualified equine physio, what advice would you give to me?

Well, I'd assume you know your medical stuff already, so I think I'd point out a few of the service-based things that are really important. You're working with people as well as horses, and to be successful you must be prepared to go the extra mile. You should show that you care, you should smile and be polite; and always try to explain everything very clearly – there's no need to be secretive or aloof. That's all to make sure you give a good service to your clients. But for your own benefit, I'd just say two things – keep bloody good records, and enjoy your job!

Very good advice, and not just for physiotherapists! I just wonder – your type of job, healing sick animals and people, is usually described as 'vocational'; but do you think that is enough to sustain someone through a long career in the health business?

Ha! Thirty years ago I would have said yes. But today? This actually came up recently when Godfrey and I were having dinner with a lovely family who all work in the NHS in roles encompassing managers, an A&E nurse and a paediatrician. With Godfrey present, the conversation always develops into a lively debate, and on this occasion it concerned their motivation for doing these jobs.

And I was really struck by their attitude – impressive, all about saving lives at any cost, protecting the vulnerable and so on - but to me at this stage in my career maybe also a little unrealistic? However I didn't want to dent their enthusiasm so instead I just told them a story.

Quite early in my NHS career I went on a management course run by a very dynamic lady who was the head of physio at Doncaster Royal Infirmary. Her first question to us was: "Why are you here today?" Now, we being young and keen – and green – we all came out with the predictable range of answers – to promote our profession, to improve our skills, to achieve world peace – and she laughed. "Bullshit," she said, "it's for the money!"

And of course she was right; physios are not well paid, so any route to promotion means more money. I'm not sure this story had much impact on our dinner friends – they are mostly on good salaries and perhaps can afford to remain more idealistic than some, but I'd love to meet them again in twenty years time and see if their optimism is still as strong.

Finally, can I just ask about your personal life? You're a real Yorkshire woman; like Godfrey you call a spade a spade – but you do have moments of real glamour and excitement in your life as well. What's that version of Katie all about?

Well, you've heard about the posh frocks, and the not-too-successful Mercedes. But I think the only real glamour actually has been some of the wonderful travelling I've enjoyed with Godfrey. Some of this came on the back of his lectures in various countries, and some of it was just our shared fascination in exploring other countries. But yes, we tend to have travelled in a degree of style – or comfort! I've enjoyed some amazing hotels: the Negresco in Nice, the Alvear Palace in Buenos Aires, Londra Palace in Venice, Brenners Park Hotel in Baaden Baaden (and if you're ever looking for a good cup of tea in Germany, that's a place I'd recommend!).

We've also had some fantastic riding holidays; gaucho horses in Argentina; basuto ponies in Zululand; rounding up cattle in Wyoming; and even riding out with an Indian Admiral in Delhi.

But it wasn't all glamour by any means. We used to visit my Grandma in Poland in the 1970s before the iron curtain was torn down. I remember being searched, counted on and off the Aeroflot plane at gun point, and knowing the KGB were always just a few steps behind wherever we went. Dad didn't help my nerves by insisting on trading his US dollars on the street rather than accepting the rip-off exchange rate in the bureaus. To be fair we did also try to redress the economic imbalance by smuggling oranges, coffee, tights and even barathea (the fabric used for making nuns' habits) across with us whenever we went.

Is there anywhere you still haven't been and want to go?

222

Yes there is – I really want to go to Portugal, and also to Russia. But I have to be honest; I think both of us are at our most excited nowadays when we've just booked a cottage holiday in Pembrokeshire for a week's walking. We've always been very keen walkers – fells, dales coastlines, and always with the dogs - and since Godfrey has had to stop riding because of back problems, we find even more time for walking - and they are very happy times indeed.

And just one last question – someone like yourself never loses their zest for life; so there must be some things out there that you still want to achieve?

I may have the zest, but I've a few war wounds too – most recently two new hips. So one thing I'd like to achieve is continued good health. But yes, I haven't hung up my stirrups just yet! I would love to do some more side-saddle riding once again. And, oh I don't know, maybe compete in a one day event – and see if see if I can get a clear round of jumping? That would be fun!

This year I have had a change of direction in the yard. I am still available for equine physiotherapy appointments, but the rehabilitation side is too much for me nowadays so it has been outsourced. I have a cottage that is available for holiday lets and am offering holidays for you and your horse or hunting holidays for you and your horse, or holidays for your horse while you go away on holiday, see wressleequestrianservices.co.uk I have some flyers/documents I will attach to see if anything can be used to help.

Katie, it's been a pleasure, thank you.

(Rupert Waddington, Editor)

Writing this book has been a roller coaster trip down memory lane. I never realized before just how many small details I had buried away – people, places and animals that had influenced my life at some point or other. Rediscovering these has sometimes been an emotional challenge, but I've laughed as well – a lot!

You see, I'm really lucky; and telling my story has reminded me just how lucky.

I was lucky to be raised by sensible parents and with sensible values. And yes, I grew up in rural Yorkshire where people are known for being tough and straightforward; but I think I have to put at least half of my industrious determination down to being half-Polish. There is as much of my eastern-European father as of my Yorkshire mother in me, and it is a blend of personalities that I feel very fortunate to have inherited.

I'm also lucky, I think, in having been born with a rebellious streak. I'm very happy to keep my head down, get stuck in and work hard, but I find it difficult not to challenge bureaucratic or puffed up nonsense. Authority where it has real purpose and is backed by simple common sense is fine. But rules just for the sake of it? Or even worse, committees whose entire focus seems to be to perpetuate their own existence? I just find it hard to let these go unchallenged. Maybe my diplomacy could sometimes have been better, but I believe in doing things for a reason, and getting them done, not just talking about them.

The last – and most valuable – piece of luck I've enjoyed was to be born with a liking for hard work. It's easy to undervalue this but I really do need to be busy – and it's this drive to be working and productive that made me determined to defy my girl's school and succeed in a professional career of my own choosing.

But of course, hard work is only half of the story; the other half is all about people, the amazing people who have had such a profound influence over my life and career.

And I must begin by mentioning an unusual bunch – the few truly awful people I've encountered through my study and work. There's something about medicine and horses that occasionally brings out the very worst in people. But their attempts over the years, deliberate or otherwise, to undermine my confidence and progress only spurred me on. So they deserve my thanks and a brief, if anonymous, mention here.

Much bigger thanks must go to the many people who have no idea just how much help they have been to me. I wish I could name them all, but often we just were ships passing in the night. When you're learning and trying out new things, you're hungry for ideas and feedback. So a brief chat here, an overheard conversation there – all these have over the years provided insight that has helped me hone my craft as a physiotherapist for man and horse. They've also helped me be a better person too, being role models for communicating and using expertise with grace and humility, and by just being really sound human beings. I thank these people from the bottom of my heart and hope you know who you are.

Medics and horse-folk can be a strange mix with even stranger sub-groups within it. One that I really must thank here are the farriers. Often undervalued, a good farrier is of the upmost importance in the horse world – "no foot, no horse"! And I have been lucky to work alongside some excellent farriers including *Phil Harland, Simon Jackson, Andy Worrall, Marc Matthison* and the amazing *Troy Owen*. A huge thank you to all of you – some owners may not realize how vital your work is but we physios certainly do!

Another sub-group (although they won't like the 'sub' part) is the hunting fraternity. Hunting has played a big part in my life since childhood. I realize that for some it is a controversial subject; if that includes you, please be reassured that my focus is on the thrills of riding and not on the techniques of pest control! So I hope this might offer a different perspective on a much-debated topic. Regardless, I certainly owe a huge debt not just to the experience that hunting has given me (more on this later in the book) but also to the world-class riders and huntsmen I've encountered while out on a meet.

The exceptional hunt riders I've encountered include *John Cottingham* and *Simon Roberts* (field masters), *Jon Roberts* (show jumper), eventers such as *Katie Stephens Grandy* and *Harriet Morris Baumber*, jockeys including *Joanna Lucy Mason*, *Jacqueline Coward* and a host of others from the Easterby/ Coward yards. It's always an inspiration and a great pleasure to see such talent in action.

While following the hunt on horseback I've also been inspired by the huntsmen who, seemingly effortlessly, keep between 24 and 32 or more hounds under control (as well as us riders). And now they also maintain hunts within the new law – truly legendary people, including amongst them *Jim Carruthers, James Bloor, William Deakin, Richard Standing, Frank Houghton Brown, Adrian Dangar, Tony Edwards, Tim Easby, Charles Carter, David Elliott, John Goode and Gareth Bow.*

In the world of equine care, one discipline stands out thanks to two exceptional practitioners – *Terry McGuiness* and *Paul Waudlby*, equine dentists. Often using manual equipment rather than the easier power tools, these skilled men both know how to work with baby and nervous horses in the most wonderful way. Rarely resorting to sedation, they nevertheless manage to give the horse a positive experience of this invasive work and boost its confidence for future treatment.

I think I'm in danger of writing the entire book in this Acknowledgements section, so instead I'd better thank other wonderful people in a list, some of whom sadly are no longer with us:

Geoff Plummer MCSP and *Alex Fuller MCSP* (Senior 1 Physiotherapists, Outpatients, Hull Royal Infirmary) – for teaching, encouraging and motivating me and giving me access to all your skills;

Mary Bromley FCSP and *Janet Ellis MCSP* – for being the original pioneering equine physiotherapists, involved in establishing ACPAT and amending the veterinary constitution;

Mrs Mary Holt – for being a legend in riding side saddle, and demonstrating so well how to ride cross country;

Mrs Sarah Sherwin – for being a marvellous side saddle teacher with a wicked sense of humour;

Bob Ordidge MRCVS, Jon Pycock MRCVS, Ieuan Pritchard MRCVS, Alistair Nelson MRCVS (deceased), Dai Davies MRCVS (deceased) and *Roddy Graham MRCVS* – for being legendary vets who I was privileged to work with and for, and for being prepared to support our techniques in the early days of equine physiotherapy. And amongst the younger vets I've worked with more recently (and who have made me feel so old) *Bryan Read MRCVS (Rainbow Equine Hospital)* and *Emma Nettleton MRCVS (Wicstun Vets);*

David Nicholson (horse seller and producer) – for great company and for producing amongst his high quality Irish horses the notable Mr Cracker who, in his later years, conveyed my husband across country until the grand age of 31;

Judi Thurloe (seller and producer) – for producing many excellent horses for purchase and as hirelings for many Yorkshire hunts, including my best ever hunter, Maestro;

Winks Green physiotherapist (South Africa) – for showing me right from the start that working with horses is a worthy but not an easy option;

A.S.Palman – for writing the inspirational book, Training Show Jumpers, which teaches simple and effective training;

Jane Collins – for being my former senior groom, rider of show horses and helping Godfrey to improve his jumping.

Jean Leighton, Sue Herd, Sandra Edmonds, Claire Swires, Heather Sharpless, Jane Corker and *Kelly 'the Saturday Girl'* – for being the lovely ladies who have helped me in the past and present looking after, producing, exercising, schooling, jumping and hunting, competing and working on all the horses that have passed through the yard as patients and private horses;

Kate Read, former assistant and rehab manager, who kept me and the business going through ill health and recovery following my hip replacements;

Ewan Elliott (Personal Trainer, Sports Massage Therapist, and Assistant Physiotherapist) – for all his patient help in the human side of the practice, building it up and now running it himself;

Rupert Waddington – for helping me organize my thoughts for the book, and tackling two new subjects – horses and physiotherapy – with gusto and perception;

My father and mother – for teaching me not to be frightened of hard work and that if you want it enough, you can achieve it!

And finally, *Godfrey* – for being there and always believing in me, and supporting guiding and, occasionally, correcting me;

But of course – let's not forget all the horses and ponies that have been loyal companions, worthy adversaries and excellent teachers across the years. Bless you all, warts 'n' all.

WRESSLE EQUESTRIAN SERVICES

Wressle Equestrian Services offers a unique place to stay not just for you but also your horse(s). Situated in Wressle, East Yorkshire, you can come and explore this beautiful part of the world enjoying peace of mind that you and your four legged friends, equine or canine, will be more than welcome.

The Vicarage Cottage provides recently modernised, Victorian era accommodation whilst the stables and the rest of the equine facilities are of the highest standard, giving you both a real 'home from home' feel and a comfortable stay.

The area provides various attractions and places of interest within close proximity with more things to do than hours in the day. Whether its history and architecture, country pursuits or coastal walks that appeal to you, we've got it all and more with a fantastic place to base your holiday from.

We also offer Hunting Holidays as well as stabling for your horse(s) if you are planning to go further afield and need them to be looked after in your absence.

More information is available on the website along with contact details.

www.wressleequestrianservices.co.uk

WRESSLE EQUESTRIAN SERVICES

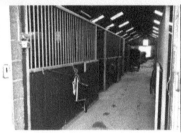
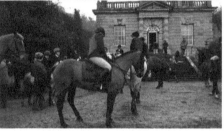

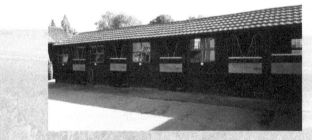

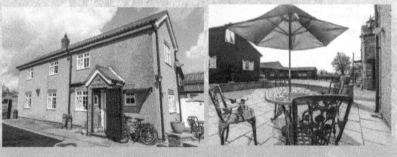

www.wressleequestrianservices.co.uk